Consciousness Since Birth

ANDROMEDA L.C.

Consciousness Since Birth

How to Feel Like the Brilliant Parent; A Healing Guide for Real People

II of III

I am Peaceful. I am Powerful. I am Purposeful.

Andromeda L.C.

ANDROMEDA L.C.

Copyright © 2018 Andromeda Limmen Chehab
All rights reserved.

No part of this book may be reproduced and transmitted in any form and by any means without the written permission of the publisher, except in the case of a few sentences used in book reviews and critical articles or presentations.

All health or medical advice should be followed up by a registered doctor. The author stands for all given advice and can not take legal responsibility for the reader's case or medical questions.

Limmen Chehab, Andromeda

First time publishing Consciousness Before Birth

First Edition

ISBN: 9781792025198

Broumanna, 2023

Distributed Worldwide

Cover design by Denis and Andromeda

Seeking design, print, bound and distribution partners

WHAT READERS SAY SO FAR

"It's Brilliant."

— Sofia Jafar, Transformational Coach

"Serious AHA-aaaaa and Yes moments!"

— Alison Bradley, Ally's Kitchen Stories

"It is a thoughtful and delightful read. Deserves to be published."

— A. J. Wallace, Editor, Economic and political work, Bahrain

WHAT CLIENTS SAY SO FAR

"Andromeda just landed in my house and pulled my head out from under the water before I drown just like a guardian angel (..) I was protected by a guardian angel. And Thank You for being that guardian angel."

- E.A.S, Client, Andromeda L.C.

"I recommend this technique (NES Health) and especially to be done through Andromeda for her mental stamina that was able to go deep down the rooted issues in my life, and was successfully able to detect milestones that was still affecting me till date. After this session I already feel relieved and made peace with the stuff that used to bother me the most, without having consciousness of it. After being brought to my awareness these things don't bother me anymore."

- N.K, Client, Andromeda L.C.

DEVOTION

I dedicate this book to all mothers out there, fighting the battle and in search of sanity and love.

I also dedicate this book to the power that is in you for being a source of love for your child, never failing them or cutting them short even when you do. You can always say "sorry", "thank you", "I love you".

Remember, words are for free. Feelings are for free. Peace is for free. Love is for free. You have access to free your mind and to free your children.

ACKNOWLEDGMENTS

I acknowledge my mother and my husband, they were both my shining examples of being more than ordinary in my epiphanies for human health (my mother) and for breaking through in spiritual and mental health (my husband) as they were the source of my darkest days and the reason for my light to keep on shining.

I can see now that they are my direct teachers of a healthy living, fulfilling relationship and enlightenment. I might have gone astray, but I've lived for a life time.

DEDICATION

I dedicate this book to Humanity.

There has been a time where people lived in peace with one another, a Garden of Eden. They were one with nature and ate from her resources as if they were eating from their own body.

When they picked an apple or a pear, they picked their eye or the eye of another to eat. The holy spirit was united with the flesh. Then a big bang of sound created a separation. We were no longer flesh of the holy spirit, we came to live in a dual world. Darkness was created and a veil held us captivated.

Now is the time to return home. Back to peace and unity. Search your soul, search your humanity. We are here to enjoy the heaven and garden which is the womb of our Mother Earth, Gaia, The All Present, The Beautiful, The Jannah of Life.

CONTENTS

1. Parenting PhD	13
2. The Friendly Intruder	30
3. Voluntary Care	34
4. Daddy Depression and Anger Management	77
5. Life Hacks	106
6. Unleashing the Tiger Mom	120
7. Peace on Earth Comes with a Peaceful Birth	175

ANDROMEDA L.C.

II of III

ANDROMEDA L.C.

1 Parenting PhD

The rumble in the jungle and your way through it

What future parents don't realize, is that it takes more than two parents to raise a child. Many relationships or broken homes evolve around one parent doing the job and they suffer from a lack of practical and emotional support. Women and men sometimes tend to the job of both mother and father; a dynamic which at least for the female ends up being too forceful, rigid and masculine in her body and mind. This build-up can certainly lead to disease and disharmony. A true harmony within a person and within a relationship is a dance between yin and yang.
I used to either feel like a single parent or too masculine every time this tendency popped up and it popped up a lot. This might go unnoticed, because in the Western society and economy it is praised for a woman to 'be like a man'

and make things work and "churn" like they do in factories. The dilemma though is that we need the feminine counterpart to "churn" at home, in families and for a warm, caring society and even companies.

There is too much work around the clock involved with caring for an infant or even an older child. They cannot or hardly be left alone a few minutes unattended. Hence the reason mothers cannot go to the toilets or take a shower. There is a total strain on the household and the feeding is practically non-stop. Provisions run out quickly and there is always something going on.

A child in return needs other family members to connect with and relate to. One caretaker, and even two, is psychology not beneficial for the child and unconsciously family units seek out a bigger "Framily" of friends and acquaintances to be an aunty or uncle to the child. The 'friendly' family members are a welcome alternative or addition to the program with children. They will also make you feel taken care of as a parent, taking a bit the pressure of the mind, or literally take care of you in a time of need.

There are different styles to choose from

When parents start wondering about "how to raise a child" there is another aspect which they might not realize at first; there are different parenting styles to choose from and make your own. These styles have been developed and described in order to subsequently make their own mix, philosophy and scope on their parent-child relationship. Being a parent is not merely about being "strict and disciplined" or "cool and friendly". There are variations to it and besides a style, you might become and remain overwhelmed by these little but undeniable creatures. When you choose your style, it will be easier to inform yourself on the chosen "PhD" and take it from there. When things are not as peaceful or disciplined as you hoped, it's time to restudy the matter and come back to it with new insights. Keep an open mind. You or your child's ways are not set in stone, especially if their behavior or your life are running off track. The last decade has been all about mindfulness and it has benefited a vast majority of people in small and big ways. I would like to bring it to the table, because it not only benefits to living your life with quality but also parenting or simply "being the parent". Parenting is therefore not so much a doing as it is a being, but "being" needs from us to be very present when our kids require our full attention for problem solving. Those windows are opportunities to set their future behavior in stone. Behaviors could be being polite, listening to your advice or instructions, self-discipline, cleaning up mess, eating without fussiness or any other behavior if you are dealing with teens.

Mindful parenting

Being mindful is about slowing down, hitting the pause button, waiting 3 seconds before speaking, meditating on your feelings and thoughts, taking new inspiration seriously, taking time out of your day to enjoy your surrounding, becoming aware of your body and spirit and eating mindfully. First of all, notice what's going on right here and right now without wanting to change it. You can repeat for your child "you are hungry", "you are hitting your brother or sister", "you said you are angry" and than take it in to process it for yourself. The more mindful you become as you practice each moment, the less judging you will be of someone else's behavior. It will get you to a point where you are not inclined or at least not urged to change it. It's human to remain somewhat inclined or urged to improve a certain situation or behavior because of your own agenda and ego. We tend to worry about the ones we care about, even if we feel they have made our lives bitter or sour with their "stubbornness". The question is; who is being stubborn?

Mindful parenting is not in order to compete in the "Olympics. of Parenting" but if there were one, you could and would be a good winner at it. Mindful parents create a safe environment for children to talk about their feelings and what they are experiencing. They also don't mind talking about their own feelings and experiences, although I want to side note that there is a realm of privacy between an adult and a child. Our children don't need to hear all the ins and outs, I believe. If you can bring the conversation delicately and gracefully, than perhaps you can share more details, but your child is not your next best friend for you to drink a glass and open up with the latest of your news. Even if it's about them. Mindful parents are or, in my eyes, should be mindful about the life, privacy and delicacy of their children's experiences. If you write one hate message or one angry letter, it might or will impact them for the rest of their lives. It would probably impact you as a parent, but then again, we are the adults and can mindfully work on our inner ego.

Mindful parents don't believe in just the good moments, they might not know all the challenges even with a helicopter view, but they know that it can be very challenging and tend to be softer on themselves as a parent and a person. Another parent, non-mindful, could fall into a child hating attitude or their own angry and fearful selves. We simply get overwhelmed and exhausted when the limit of the day or week is reached or all our buttons are pushed. The same goes for a child though. Them too get overwhelmed, exhausted and beyond limits. Just imagine how life is with you as a parent and what your are telling them and making them do all day and all week long. They have an incredible amount of information and personal information to process besides their bodily sensations like sleep, hunger, sadness, anger. A mindful parent will sense when their patience is running thin and to step away and plan in that necessary break or get the professional help to sort things out. Often we need someone to help us with that last push though.

Different Mindful Parenting Styles
- Continuum Concept
- Gentle Parenting
- Peaceful Parenting
- Attachment Parenting (John and Mary)
- Aware Parenting
- Conscious Parenting
- Mindful Parenting
- Whole-brain parenting

Attachment is the glue of a relationship

A healthy attachment goes both direction and means: acceptance of the other's reactions, concern for emotional and physical wellbeing of the other, interest in the hobbies and (school) education of the other.

An unhealthy attachment means that either the child, parent or partner is no longer interested in the wellbeing of the other, they are neglected, hated or left behind.

Did you know it is possible to have an attachment break with your parents, even if you have lived with them practically your whole life? There tends to be an attachment break if you cannot accept the reactions of another.

Besides the overall attachment there can be a lack of empathy created between the two individuals, especially in an authoritative relationship. When a parent does not display empathy to a child, there is an attachment break and the child will not have reason to care about the feelings of the parent. They will rather care about your reactions and rules. Rules and reactions become more important than respect. If we don't give respect to our child from early on, we cannot expect to have respect in return. The relationship becomes rather superficial and complex. The same can happen between a boss or manager and their employees. In companies there is also a parental relationship and taking care of the employees can be considered parenting. The employee will feel this relationship more directly because they are in a more vulnerable position. The same counts for our children. We will take a deeper look at this in the context of unconscious parenting.

What happens if we are unconsciously parenting?

First of all there tends to be shouting, commanding, demanding, bargaining and manipulating. Sounds like a toddler or teenager to you? You have guessed wrong. I welcome you to the creature called a parent. Isn't it the parents constantly shouting, commanding, demanding, bargaining and manipulating or simply denying the child's existence?

The parent misses out on the opportunities that the child presents you to have:

1. A composed, controlled and healthy behavior inside and outside of the home
2. A cooperation and relationship with your child that you (and your child) enjoy
3. A steady path to a happy childhood and successful adult life for your child and remaining in connection with your children
4. Your child will be an aware individual and more conscious on life in a broad sense, more skilled to control body and mind, have more self-confidence and be more capable of controlling his/her life's creations

To have a healthy attachment with your child, it is extremely important to establish this in the first year of life: the Diamond Year. The year where it all happens, the year where we make it or break it. This is the foundation we set in stone for our child's life. This is what they will know and put on repeat. If there was no attachment because of physical separation, no quality time, no evolvement in tender, loving, care, than we are destined for an unhealthy attachment. No matter the situation you were in or the excuses, the baby has started out life in an unattached way which will continue to be its existence, especially on a soul level. We store all our physical and emotional memories in our cells of our body and although our brains are flexible and our hearts are forgiving, it is very hard for the "hardware" to change. The software can be updated, but the hardware is kind of there. This is why the Continuum Concept and Attachment Parenting debate for an continues attachment in the beginning of baby's life until they have become more independent.

Some research describes the styles of attachment as either secure, avoidant or anxious. As everyone has a certain type of being attached to this world, you will have one of these three styles and start relating to other people and your romantic partner in this same corresponding way. We learn about intimate and romantic relationships from the place you least expect it: from the parents.

Is it not a shame if your children were to fall into the category of anxious or avoiding? You make the difference to the rest of their lives and prevent the suffering that perhaps you have seen in your (grand)parents and within yourself.

Attachment as a base for happiness

An unhealthy attachment is called an Attachment Disorder or Reactive Attachment Disorder (RAD). This might also be the base of ADHD. AD/RAD can manifest in different ways but the main way is that baby, child or teen does not trust the caregivers which makes his caregiving environment to be there for him for whatever he needs. I also believe that the parent can have the attachment disorder towards the child rather than the child towards the parent, even if the parent has held the baby in a carrier most of the time. A parent can feel like they failed their child or they went through such a hard time, they cannot separate their anxiety from their child. Perhaps they are still suffering of postpartum depression, a traumatic birth or a traumatized marriage and pregnancy. Perhaps the Attachment Disorder can set in at a later stage of the child's life, but still relate to the original trauma and disconnect from the parent. Whatever the cause might be; the parents don't feel attached or a likeness towards the child. They might feel not liked or loved by that particular child, although the child does love, but in their own particular way or with a misunderstanding which needs to be cleared out by communication. How well do you know your child on a personal level? Have you discussed your feelings with them, no matter their age, in order to know more about their fragile lives? Have you tried to clear out the air? I had a attachment situation with my 4 year old and so I decided to clear it out over several two-way conversations, which made us find the attachment for both to express ourselves more authentically, wether the ideas were negative or positive.

With an attachment disorder we will observe and experience, most likely, all of the behaviors below throughout their young years and adult years:

- Behaving inappropriately in social situations
- Wondering: what is going on in the child?
- Have difficulty trusting the child and vice versa
- Have difficulty with peers
- Difficulty with attention or behavior
- Disrupted development
- Aggressive or explosive reactions

- An inward, autistic or borderline personality
- Depression, suicidal, addictions
- Unhappy intimate relationships
- Not much stability or sustainability

Other factors that contribute to RAD: baby loses his caregiver, illness of the mother, parent not available emotionally, unpredictable caregiving, abuse and neglect. These events and treatments show up in the structure of the brain, particularly in case of neglect. The rice experiment by Dr. Emoto is a great proof of the damaging effect of emotional neglect, even more than hate. We will discover this later on in the book.

The regulation of fears are affected by Attachment Disorders; they set off, they explode. As an outsider you might not see which need exactly is not met, which one sets them off and their reaction might be scare you, but it is their survival to overreact. It's like tantrums and usually hunger, sleep, needs and wants are a trigger. You can see the same dynamic within any type of partner or within an intimate relationship like a marriage.

With all these new concepts and terms mentioned in this book, I advice you to do your further research through articles and videos online as well offline with books and conversations with professionals and other parents, until you find yourself well-rounded on the general subject. Make your own conclusions and follow your instinct of what is the source and solution for your baby, because otherwise society will tell you. If a subject affects you and your child directly, it's extra sensitive to our mind, ego, insecurities and emotions. These experiences give you an opportunity for your consciousness about body, mind and soul to expand

On another side note, RAD might be seen or diagnosed as bipolar, add, hyperactivity and perhaps autism but these and RAD are never resolved if treated solely with medications. Autism or true autism, not merely an introverted personality, or other modern day ailments need to be treated with a severe detox through nutrition, diet, homeopathy, fresh oxygen, blood regeneration and other treatments that contribute to detoxing from harmful vaccinations and pollution through medication, environment and diet. The initial toxic can be provoked by vaccinations, if you had an infant that was fine prior to vaccinations and changed their reactions, especially after a booster.

You might see parenting as time consuming and a loss of energy when it is tender, loving and caring towards your children, but research, science and personal experiences show the opposite to be true if you seek happiness for yourself and for your children. You are inseparable in your inner-experiences.

Parenting through the decades

The 50's Parenting: Discipline, clock work, routine, don't touch baby, separate room, no touch and no-eye contact, bottle fed is easier, Truby King Method. Ruled by parents of the post-war era.

The 60's Parenting: Baby love, free lifestyle for the parents, attended to baby on baby's cues, moses baskets, must not feel guilt if not breastfeeding, day care starts, Benjamin Spock. Ruled by parents of the working class families.

The 70's Parenting: Tribal, constant contact first 6 months, total inclusion, co-sleeping, breastfeeding on demand, the Continuum Concept. Ruled by parents of the hippies lifestyle.

The 80's Parenting: Dr. Spock "the bible" revival, babies don't have a watch, balancing between discipline and free reign, "independence" above all, economics above all, brands and corporations, white coats became authority. Ruled by parents of The American Dream.

The 90's Parenting: pop-culture, outdoors, camping, adventures, travel, road trips, arts and crafts, second hand clothing, colorful, bold expressions, free style, care free, family life, family values, creativity above economics, games and gaming, entertainment above all, career oriented, success and skills, new age movement, practical foods, candy. Ruled by the parents of Pop.

21st Century Parenting: internet revolution, news and media revolution, individual expression, overprotective, helicopter parenting, money driven parents, business owners, being my own business, millennial generation, personal branding, modern day ailments or disease, underfed, toxic, unseen challenges in the world, terrorism, wars, war on religion, technology instead of bond, addicted, social media values, information age, freedom, lost, materialistic, egocentric, isolated, personal responsibility, self-esteem and confidence above all, coaching and therapies become mainstream, seeking humanity, interest in holistic health, clean nutrition movement, seeking natural, seeking basic human nature, spiritual revival.

The Current Parenting: becoming a coach to your child and being a communicator is the main pillar of the modern day parenting. It is up to you to find how you can sooth your child no matter what age, by asking them what they need or want, practicing anger and stress management, becoming independent and self-reliable, focusing on personal responsibility, taking motherhood and fatherhood as a priority, keeping open and direct communication, work on interpersonal skills, such as emotional intelligence, solving conflicts, making heartfelt connections, giving emotional freedom, letting space for self-expression, embracing total acceptance, letting unconditional love take over ego, setting up foundations for future love relationships. Also, parenting is openly discussed with others in the community without taboos. A parent must make it a mission to find Inner Peace to find a peaceful existence in a highly complicated and sensitive world where past influences are built on generations and decades of "bad parenting".

The Future Parenting: parenting in a community, tribal living, shared wisdom, natural healing, respected approach, sustainable, from the source, environmental friendly, we are soul seekers, star people, inter dimensional, Peace is on Earth.

So how can you parent in a positive way that fits today's norms as described above?

By being a coach and guide to your child, you can start to parent from a respectful source instead of the authority of disrespect. Seeing, hearing and listening to your child's needs is a first stip. By practicing "Living in the Now", "Slowing Down", "Having Fun" and "Being Soft on One-Self" we become a more happy, peaceful parent from within and fitting ourselves into the daily routines and rhythms. By looking for calm, confident and compassionate attitudes within yourself and your children you and your children become calm, confident and compassionate. By fostering long term relationships with your children, you find partners for life with peace, power and purpose. These are some of the things to look for in your daily attention, attitude and approach.

This article and forum describes modern day parenting and, to my consideration, what conscious parenting embodies. I am happy to dedicate a the end of this chapter to echoing what Emem Nwogwugwu, the Project Manager of La Pax Nigeria, speaks, advocates and writes about through the forum 'Let's Chat Moms' on the challenges of modern day parenting:

"We are not coming to raise perfect kids. There is no such thing as perfect human beings. We want kids who have empathy and a sense of responsibility in their lives and their environment. We want kids who will own their actions and be responsible for their decisions in life, people who understand consequences and benefits, people who have a balanced way of thinking."

"We are here because of love. The world needs love. Despite the parental competition in the world, we are hoping to bring up balanced confident and loving people who will be faithful leaders of tomorrow, who will shine their lights in areas where there is darkness and kids who will learn how to forgive because they will need that on their inter-personal relationship journey now and in the future. We want to be better, we want to network with like minds to reach a common global goal of raising excellent examples in all aspects of life, now and in the future."

Other mothers who also made inputs at the forum were of the view that children are special gifts and each child has a talent and how it is harnessed is entirely dependent on the parent, whether the child is physically challenged or not. They explained further that there was a window of between 0-3 years and 3-6 years and that these periods were when the core values and foundations are built in children, as it was also the periods that are easiest to assist with any developmental challenges a child may have.

The mothers particularly stressed on the fact that parents should examine what kind of parents they were, which will help also in determining how they can relate with their children and confront difficulties they may exhibit, adding that parenting style also has a huge influence on how a child behaves or confronts different situations.

"They need to learn about conflict resolution, how to manage their anger and other things that they need to deal with people in the world basically because in these days and age, it is not enough to learn just ABC, if you don't have good inter-personal skills you can't even work anywhere."

"Montessori education is very important to me because it teaches children independence and independence is something that we really need for our children because with that children are able to think for themselves, they are able to think creatively and they are able to think practically as well. When they have independence, they are not going to wait for people to help them do things always, but can do things themselves and this gives them a lot of confidence and self-esteem and for me that is the most important thing that a child needs to have so that as they grow up to adulthood, they would still maintain that self-esteem and confidence to do whatever they want to and also to face the world and conquer it."

The Science of Parenting; there is no such thing! Yet, there is so much to learn, keep an open mind.

- Andromeda L.C.

2 The Friendly Intruder

Getting to know your baby as an actual person

You've been two individuals, you formed a couple and you were getting along so far. Now, post-partum, you are not just an extra individual - you are heading for a family life. This is the one reason of how and why life will change forever and ever.

What is a family? What is family life? This concept has absolutely no correlation to your previous couple life. Now that your baby has arrived you are building a fort, slowly and surely you might or most likely will experience a sequence of attacks on your fort.

The fort could break down and crumble to ruble, or it can stand strong, each time rebuilt from its foundation. Or it could be some kind of ruin and visited by seasonal tourists. Are you going to rebuild your fort? Or do you choose to desert it and find new grounds to stand your guard? It's a choice and sometimes the war is bigger than ourselves. The couple might have been strong, but they were protected in an ivory tower before the arrival of the friendly intruder. A family is about coming down to Earth and building new walls on the foundation of the couple's strengths and family values that live from within. If the foundation was not great to begin with, it still has to be built one way or another because your child is now the ivory tower and must be guarded, whatsoever.

I consider it a crime to let a child break down to Earth, if it is our job to try our utmost, through process of birth, to bring the child back to the Heavens. The intruder, the baby that is born into the couple, will probably make the whole foundation shake. Especially if the father or mother will experience the new individual as an intruder; he or she is taking away all the time and attention of the previous girlfriend or boyfriend. Being a parent and a partner is far from easy. We need to know what it means to 'create a new life'.

The mother has carried the seed of life in her belly for nine months, but was not acquainted to the actual friendliness or unfriendliness of the intruder into her life. She was aware of being pregnant and her body changing accordingly, she was not aware of the person living in her and their midst.

When the baby is a boy, he becomes competition to daddy. When the baby is a girl, mommy feels the competition with her daughter, especially towards daddy and might become extremely jealous in the process. Why is the baby girl getting Daddy's sweet love? Where is this love for me? He used to once give me attention but it is long gone now. Does he love the baby girl like he loves me? Does he love the baby more than me? And in the same manner, the baby girl or boy can grow jealous of the same sex parent, because they know their parent is married and belongs to the couple, not to them. This is called the Oedipal complex. Being an authentic parent requires maturity.

We all love babies in different ways, and we love a baby in a different way than we love our partner. I think that is the most reasonable conclusion. It remains utterly personal and it is our personal responsibility to make it work.

This chapter was the shortest, yet it has the most impact on your new life and measures the success or the failure of your marriage and more importantly: family life. Your individual expression is part of a bigger thing. This could make it or break it.
What if the child is different from you? What if the child doesn't have the same looks as you? What if the child is disabled, sick or ill? What if the character and interests are totally not you? Can you accept this person in your midst? Can you start to believe that this also is part of you? That every child reflects a part of the parent's being or legacy? That even an odd child is part of your love, hobbies and interests? Each child reflects an individual aspect of your being and you as a parent are the whole of it. Only you have

the power to empower your child with LOVE, especially the first year of life and with some corrections and compensations from your side during the Early Childhood if needed, so "later" when they are teenagers and young adults you can foster and enjoy a life and a shared relationship. Than I guess the rest, "they will do pretty much on their own" as they say. Good luck!

3 Voluntary Care

Who will take care of the baby and you? The challenges of being a mom and a parent at the same time

You can decide for yourself, to take on being a mom as a full-time profession, but be careful how you balance your new life. This means, you will dedicate your time and efforts to the full-time job, yet you require compensation. Being a full-time mom requires the same, specific skills as any other career to make it successfully through the day, week, month, year. The responsibilities are tremendous. Not only caring for your child single handedly so many hours of the day, but also to deal with your own self-care and life with extremely limited resources. The personal challenges are not few and overall moms seems to be challenged, more by the spiritual baggage than the practical care. You wonder how so many parents get through the day safe and sane.

When you talk with other parents they tend to confess that they feel like they won't make it through another day, week, month, year. I was there too and still until today. Parents are about to lose their sanity. Unfortunately there is no pay and the level of personal respect for the mom job from yourself and others is particularly low. The absence of colleagues will leave you in a solitude that seems to last forever. Slowly your old identity chips and fades away to be left with only your old troubles. If not quickly replaced by a meaningful, positive new attitude in your mom-life, you can find yourself struggling to rebuild your new self. Your new self is washed down by all the problems you are facing and the challenges ahead. You try to fight the idea that this is really "it" and seek out the solutions to get your social and work life involved in your mom-life. Once you are able to lose your ego and step into the selflessness the mom hood really is, you have set a foundation for a new, constructive self and sustainable family life. You are a nobody and now, in that void you have the chance to become yourself. A self with a heart. Your old ego and past life has been completely chipped off and stripped down to its remains.

> *The Phoenix rises from its ashes*

Challenges of the SAHM

What are some of the challenges of the SAHM: stay-at-home-mom? And why necessarily a SAHM? Not for the reason of "having no time", because everyone already had time. For the reason that during the working hours she is taking care of her children, which she considers work, as it is hard and tedious work, and she doesn't get a physical separation from her children let alone a break on her own when the evening hits. Fortunately or unfortunately, working moms will need to consider that their job time is a big "me-time", because of physical separations from kids and working on the self. These are two major things SAHM does not get and which makes it very hard to be a "full on mom". Not saying, that being a full on mom is a healthy balance, because we all need a balance between home, rest and career; it's all work for that matter. The society doesn't allow much division between part-time working mom and part-time working dads. Either time doesn't allow it or financials don't allow it, so in all cases we tend to be stuck unless we have creative solutions to our problems. The trend these times are for moms to become mompreneurs, which means they open a business to combine their passion, finance and baby at the same time. Usually it starts out as a one-man show or it involves the help of family members, but it could be a bigger enterprise or franchise that sustains the family and which allows flexible office times and locations. Anything is possible, it requires usually the same or stronger dedication as a regular job at an employer, but you are self-made in an entrepreneurial kind of way. The moms find themselves overworking and overthinking their business as well the challenge of combining the baby's schedule with their own life is still very challenging and you might still be stuck to the home. Back to SAHMs!

The Challenges:

- taking time for themselves in the home
- taking time for themselves out of the home
- taking time with or for their friendships
- taking time for intellectual development and earning money despite no job
- taking time for exercise to keep physically and mentally fit
- taking time to be physically separated from her children to recuperate

Like any high performance job, the SAHM needs to be physically and emotionally available for their children all day and every day. The intensity of the job due to the extension of her life with another fragile life along with the psychological and daily challenges, make the job feel like the hardest job on the planet. The SAHM needs another physical and creative outlet in order to stay fit. A physical outlet like walking, running, swimming, yoga, horse riding or anything else, will give the mind and spirit a break of the otherwise tiring routine. I have not been a shining example in the physical exercise department, as many moms with me, as we often fail in taking time or being disciplined for our wellbeing. I believe though it is probably the one thing that can give a mom me-time, an energizer and time with others, all in one. Some classes provide a mommy and baby postnatal workout or yoga. Yoga at home or with a personal trainer is also a possibility, although it gives the desired physical result, it will mean you are missing out on the social contact with other moms and babies.

I didn't feel physically energized for the first year. I was at the swimming pool, doing laps, stretching my legs at home or dancing in the kitchen. Did I meet anyone by doing that? Did I reduce my loneliness in the mom-hood? Did I reduce the stress of a social brain? Was I a better person or mother because of it? No. It worked for me to not commit to a place and time, but it is great if you can make it to classes and meet a group of other young mothers to share the experience and build lifelong friendships. The babies can grow up together and go on play dates to each other's houses. It ticks so many boxes, and most importantly for our brains to associate with other adults and connect on a different level. Our brain truly is a social brain. It needs physical presence of groups in order to survive. Without the social context, we die off.

I started organizing Mommy's Playdates where moms meet informally and babies play, trough these meet ups I have made some awesome friendships. I acknowledge the physical stress of the mom job. It becomes so much less stressful on a personal level, when we can share our time and resources with other women and children. Unfortunately, we often live in very isolated cubicles, called houses. This is why it is important to find some sense of community, play groups or a circle of mom friends, in order to solve many of the problems you experience in practical life, in your mind and with your children. Other moms might have the right solution for you, take of the pressure and share the same problems. As a matter of fact, you have the right to have not only time with your friends, but to have regular meet ups with your colleagues which are the other moms. Colleagues? Yes, of course! Other moms share the same vision and goals and you need to exchange all the ins and outs on how to handle the goals and obstacles. It is absolutely no luxury to spend as much time as you can afford, surrounded by people or at other homes and places.

Phoenix rising

I felt really uncomfortable with the experience of being forced into an unbalanced life act and it remains to this day a problem of balancing out me-time. During periods of extreme fatigue, the me-time is just a pause from the children and keeping my health and sanity. Once the extreme fatigue has passed and the body's balance postpartum is back into swing, the me-time becomes another job. We all have a desire to be working and productive. Unfortunately the mom-job, no matter how intense, productive and consuming, it doesn't reach the level of the kind of job we seek. It is missing the social element of contributing within a group or a platform and there is hardly or no reward. A job in the market, based on a salary, becomes the necessary me-time. Unless some Scandinavian societies people don't consider raising your baby or child as a job on its own. Not only that, you will miss out on career and pension plan as well as other benefits. Perhaps even a car to get around, which was my case as an account manager. Besides, you are not creating any savings. This is when marriage kicks in or should kick in. To prevent future issues I wished, and kind of asked, my husband to understand the day I would become a full time mom I wouldn't have any income. This question arose during some meetings with an accountant and I realized the threat and weak position of me as a wife investing all her energy and time in creating a family instead of a career or savings. He didn't see the point of that as we have an account in common and he felt it as his responsibility to provide the income being the husband. That was a big deal for him and weighed heavily on his shoulders. Especially considering he quit the project three months after our baby was born and was in between jobs for six months. Besides that, he thought it would still be feasible for me to make money any time during or after the maternity leave. He kept asking and pressuring this point with me. This was a big shock to me. How am I expected to make any kind of money while being sick or taking care of a baby? Helpless.

Marriage with children

I was clearly not going to keep my baby full-time in a creche, maximum 1 day per week or 2 afternoons until a later stage. Later I realized these expectations and disappointments I was confronted with by my husband were a part of reality of being a woman and a mother as well part of the daddy depression. I still don't consider our situation normal, but strong emotions don't usually have a logic explanation. And becoming a parent is more shocking for a couple than we can see from the outside world. So I assume that all or most couples struggle with this equation but to different degrees. I believe I was in the worst of class. Considering the percentage of divorce after the first baby, this possibility shouldn't come to us as a surprise. Unfortunately it's usually the woman and mother that suffers from the consequences, especially if there is a (future) separation. In the best cases the marriage is in her favor and the father will be obliged by law to financially contribute and take part time care of the children. If the law fails and the father flees from parenthood, she will be left taking care of the children and finances alone. Most women from failed marriages will go back to their parents for this reason and find a new partner that can contribute sufficiently on finances sooner or later. This was a common picture in the 80's and 90's and perhaps less the attitude nowadays because women are not willing to sacrifice themselves in yet another relationship and lose there emotional independence when being single and financially free. Kids need their moms at the end of the day. Women expect the father to take on his responsibilities towards his children and towards her before, during and after marriage, but this is not always or usually not the case. The law is not always strong enough to keep the cashflow ongoing from the father towards his children or wife. Whatever the situation, the majority of women will keep sacrificing her career or any means of income before, during and after marriage with children. This is not to speak about the enormous drama and threats that come with divorce. The relationship just is not over yet, it continues as it was, but through a separation.

Financial Freedom

Was I able to go to a job or make money? Was I able to find a nursery, family member or other babysitter? For financial freedom I needed baby freedom, which means someone else is taking care of the baby for all my absent minutes of the day. There was no family member around to help out. And certainly no reliable ones that had the comforting connection with a baby. I tried the creche 2-3 days per week. I brought the baby after he woke up from his morning nap around 11.30 am. I picked him up between 5-6 pm and never realized the true reality of what a creche is until I was doing it, half-baked. It means: disposing your tiny and needy baby early in the morning before traffic jam starts and picking him up after traffic jam ends just in time for the creche to close. This means that your tiny baby is taken care of by professionals for 12+ hours, most of it crying, staring or playing with plastic toys. I thought my first baby (three months old) was fine at the creche; he didn't mind me handing him over to the caretakers and didn't seem to cry. The caretaker gave me the feedback each day: they held him in the arms all day, he didn't want to be put down into a seat. Smart baby. He had only been quiet if he was in her arms, didn't drink his bottles and slept maximum 20 minutes of the whole day. Stressed baby. Was he supposed to go to the creche every day to settle into the routine? Is the creche too clinical and run by strangers? Or was he too aware of his surroundings and other babies were by comparison more acceptant of their faith? Was I spending too much time with my baby, spoiling him and myself?

As I brought him home, on every occasion he drank unlimited milk and slept directly. Hungry and exhausted baby. The following three days he was out of his usual routine and sassiness at home. Unbalanced baby. Then I brought him again to the creche according to schedule. It's a pleasure for the mom to be liberated of the burden and the exhausting job of being a mom. Relieved mom. It's a pleasure for the mom to go to work and have her 'normal' life back, whatever the job is about. Joyful mom. And even if your job became less of a priority, it's a place to breath and reset the mind. Unstressed mom. It's not wonderful being responsible all day of your baby and it's not wonderful for a baby of a working mom to spend all his days in the creche. What to do?

To creche or not to creche

The first 6 months up to one year of age are what I call the Diamond Year. You are laying the foundation of the babies physical, mental and emotional health. He is attached to you in all aspects and in full development of his brain, body and confidence in the world we live in. A baby that stays home with mom, actually doesn't really stay home with mom and become an unsocial being. Mom goes to the city, to the supermarket, receives or visits her friends, takes baby on discovery tours, visits museums and parks and visits baby classes. A baby in the creche remains with the same group of people between the same walls, every single day.
What are you giving your three month old when he goes to a creche? What love, nurture and stability does a baby receive from a caretaker? How is the baby learning about structure, confidence, trust, development? Everything the diamond shaping year is about, in my opinion, is not practisized in the creche. The competences in the Diamond Year are given from the moment we are in this life until we gradually become more independent as a 1 year old. Life doesn't start in the second year or when you think the child is to be taken more seriously. Our life and our inner wellbe-

ing starts at day 0. If you were miserable most of the time in year 1 you will be miserable in year 21 and adulthood.

Do you really think a sterile environment can provide the competences needed for full development? If you don't want to be a full-time or part-time mom until 6 months of age, than reconsider if you have the will and the time to have children. Besides that a baby of 0-6 months is as vulnerable as anyone could ever be. Neither talking, nor walking, constantly feeling needy, hungry and especially sleeping are his main tasks in life. But is the creche set up for sleeping? Or is there constant noise, distractions and stress of all sorts?

The baby needs his crib, his bottle and his mommy, more than anything else especially up to month 6-7 when they start weaning and discovering the world outside of the house. Baby doesn't need to play at this age. In fact, they don't have the actual skill to play socially with other children until the age of 4-6 years old. They are mainly growing, developing and observing through their caretaker. Besides the feeding and sleeping the baby needs to bond, bond and bond again with one or two caretakers. He doesn't need an alarm at 6 am and a long wait in his chair until 6pm, being attended to by strangers and waiting on his faith. Neither does he need to be stimulated or disturbed by other children who are older and running around and sometimes touching or boxing his face. I'm not inclining that staying with an overstressed mom is the ultimate solution, because a creche might be the ultimate safe and structured place. Although there are also negative school environments and school owners, similar and worse to the one I signed up my baby.

There is a lot to be said about why or why not a creche. There is limited scientific research to answer this question. The best answer is to imagine yourself as the baby. And second, to follow your gut, your reasoning and reevaluation each three months. An evaluation can tell you what to do next. It will depend on you as a mom if you can do the job of a solitude mom for the time being or if you need or want to search other solutions in life.

What do you really, really want for your baby? Remember, it's only a phase, perhaps a phase of sacrifice for six months in case you raise the baby from home until that age. And what do you believe in more, opposed to what society tells you to do? Be bold in your decision. Don't go mainstream. Don't think other people got it right when they say the creche is normal and a stay-at-home mom is not. Or the other way around! Don't be fooled that you really need the money more than your baby needs you up to 6-7 months of age. This is when baby starts to sit and crawl which makes him so much more independent in the creche and more flexible to move around and start the beginnings of play. Your baby will have had the chance to grow his confidence and self-worth, which he would otherwise miss. You are the one that can decide to be your baby's caretaker and for how long, until you divide your time with another family member, friend, professional or paid force. You have the right and a human need to have time off from your baby. This is something I absolutely missed in the first year and even more so in the proceeding years, although I ended up finding a routine for my elder baby when I was pregnant and nurturing the second.

Which choices to make

The first choice is having a baby, the second choice is your parenting belief and the third choice is: who is going to take care of the baby? In the beginning you'll be more needy and support is undeniable, especially in the first 1/2 year. It makes you wonder about the balance in the second year, the third year and so on? Until kindergarten or school comes around to take over a chunk of the day. But don't be fooled, school schedules don't allow a parent to work 9-6 pm and even if you use the before and after school babysitting services on a daily basis the pickup remains at 6 pm sharp. Financially as well as emotionally you will feel the impact of the (im)possibilities. So there is a lot to figure out on this matter and with a second baby there is no copy paste situation because you have to fit in the schedule of the second with the schedule of the first. Usually, this is where grandparents kick in. But with the modern nomadic lifestyle, you as an individual and society need a more creative and community approach to child-caring. In the end, every family unit finds their way around this issue and from problematic situations can come new possibilities, new friendships, new mommy businesses and more.

Parenting is a semi full-time job, because full-time is nearly to physically impossible. I've been there. I've done it and it wasn't funny. If it is not your thing to parent semi full-time then I want to encourage you to still take care of your baby until 6-7 months of age and still look for an equilibrium between home-time and creche-time. Not for any particular reason, except the fact that a baby in it's first year is a physical fragile being in a full blown developmental phase. Also, the baby's mind and soul is answering the questions: Am I lovable? Am I safe? If this is answered positively there is a positive attachment to life and the world. If not, there is a problem for life. This Diamond Year is a year where the baby diamond is:

- Small, Fragile, Sensitive, Handicapped
- Developing his inner world and bonding with outside world and people
- Developing brain capacity and linking neurons
- Developing senses
- Developing trust, confidence and safety
- Developing social skills
- Developing personal skills
- Has no spoken language

Also, as this book conveys, there is full potential in the first year to build a solid foundation for life. No gaps. The only chance for YOU to develop with your baby and to be on top of it, is for you to be there: on top of the job.

The baby depends 100% on it's mother in the first year. Let that sink in. The baby is 100% dependant on you . Until the second or even third year the child cannot be co-dependant on him- or herself. The mother or main caretakers could be careless, abusive or too ill to take on the job, surely a professional or an adoptive parent should take over in those cases.

What would you choose if you were a baby: "work" or home?

Home being your house and your mother's:
- Devoted, undivided help
- Attention
- Special, personalized care
- Warmth of home
- Your bed
- Your products and smells
- No screeches and noise
- Undisturbed sleep
- Cuddles

"Work" being a sterile environment or stranger's:
- Shared, group focus
- Superficial, general care
- Not your home, away from home
- Shared seats and beds
- Screeches and noise
- Multiple caretakers
- Noisy and crowded
- Helpless if not heard

When there is one lady taking care of 7-8 children in her home or even your child only, you should consider that you have a hard time doing that job, so why would she be able to keep it up peacefully? She's regulated by law, but she'll be doing the job in her personal space and by herself at most times. The advantage is having the personal ambiance and relationship between your baby and the "2nd mother". The disadvantage being that the job is not shared unless there are two women or a father teaming up to take care of the baby diamond. Imagine yourself 5 days per week with 7-8 babies and you'll get the picture. Nonetheless, these are usually very experienced women and there are moms very content with this solution and maybe even more content with than a professional daycare solution. You can look into other personal solutions for the baby's first year, like, a child-minder, au pair, nanny, aunt to share the job with you. Personally I haven't come around to that solution and I cannot let go of a full-time responsibility and attachment in the first 9 months of life where baby is attaching to me and at the same time letting go of me in the second half of the year.

First half year:

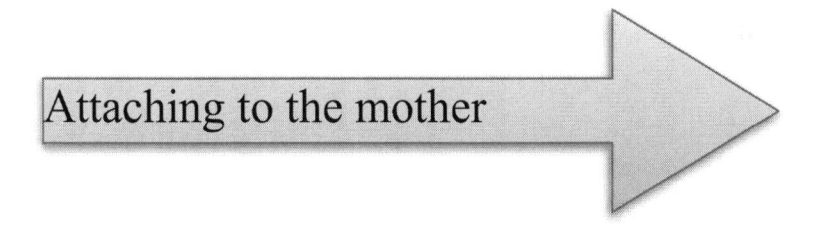

➡ Attaching to the mother

I wouldn't want the burden of (my) baby on one caretaker. And if it is at a stranger's house, you will never know which other family members or guests pass by their house. Like I said, there is a lot to figure out for your personal situation and it's a touchy subject when it comes down to your own children.

Second half year:

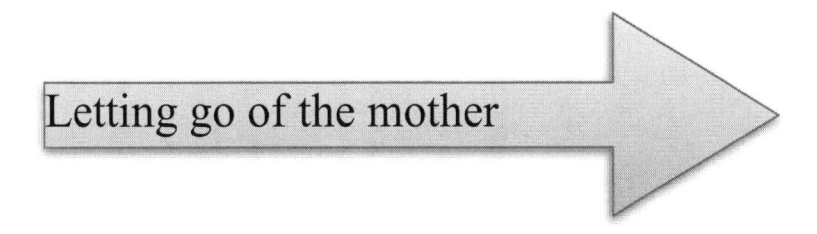

➡ Letting go of the mother

After 6-7 months passed

When the baby reaches 6-7 months, they are more solid, they can sit and they had an adjustment period of 6-7 months to the exterior world versus the mother's womb.

After 7 months, sooner or later, a baby will start crawling. In the same week the baby starts crawling, it transitioned from being a helpless baby to a scavenger. In this stage baby will start discovering the house, touching all items and playing somewhat independently. Even if he's not interested in his toys, he is interested in electrical appliances. Your role will diminish a slight bit to the background. The baby is physically more resistant, has developed senses, has a confidence to get a message across to a stranger, can impose his will, and all of this without even really talking.

Personally I believe my baby should be walking, before it's ready to go without mommy to a daycare. Part of that reason being the way daycares are set up. The creche is not at all quiet, peaceful and cosy like a baby's bedroom. They could be! If the daycare would be focused on the babies physical sensitivity to sight, sound and touch, but most often the day care are an open area plan with the toddlers and babies mixed. They are sat on the cold ground and left to wait in their rocking seats for the majority of the day.

When the baby can walk, it means they are ready for an introduction into tot and toddler activities, like strolling around, climbing, dollhouses, crafts, dancing etc. As a toddler they become more interested in children of their own age but they cannot play together. As a parent, you won't be able to provide the activities and settings, so you will start feeling this shortcoming. Even a playgroup doesn't provide the structure, group feeling and routine of a daycare. And I hardly think you will spend 8 hours per day at a playgroup.

When your toddler is talking, it means they can make themselves somewhat more heard at the daycare and they can report their day to the parents including their experiences and emotions. But talking doesn't usually come until much later than for many first children. Speech will appear between 1,5 - 3,5 years of age.

If your child is not ready for the daycare, your child might be facing distress, boredom, tuning out, apathy. A more careful build up can give your child a chance to grow into the environment and structure of a daycare. Instead of a full-time schedule your child could go to the creche 3 mornings or afternoons per week or 2 full days per week. Recommended for sensitive babies is to have sequenced days, otherwise your baby will never adapt and is switching constantly between two environments.

To creche or not to creche, that's the question

Taking care of your own child is considered the hardest job in the world. It's a task that consumes you in a physical, mental and emotional sense. Your baby is an extension of you that is fully dependant and later on co-dependant on you up to age four. I mention age 4 because up to that age, they are still overstimulated by being in a school setting and they will need your physical and emotional attention in order to rebalance their day and ideally to grow up in physical, emotional and mental stability. There is some research and literature needed here, but this is based on my observations.

The daunting task of mothers have made them vulnerable and prone to become chronically depressed or bitter. Especially with a history of depression in the family, we become more prone to developing or provoking what lies in family patterns. Nowadays, women want to stay healthy, vibrant and personally fulfilling, so accepting a depressed or bitter life is almost out of the question. Most mothers have gruesome thoughts of being like their own mother. So we set a path to do some things the same and some things differently, in order to fill in the gaps. Eventually we can tune out our own complexes and those of the previous generation of women that we didn't heal (yet).

> **The mother tiger doesn't stay small. She becomes older and wiser, changes shapes, shifts through reality, and becomes a faint expression of what life used to be. - Andromeda L.C.**

Whatever the situation, you are going to feel the weight on your shoulders and mind in the mornings, evenings and nights. The chance to go to your job will feel like a relief instead of work, because caring for a baby is far harder of a job. The intensity of tasks that need to be done to watch your baby are more intense compared to a professional caretaker, because of the emotional relationship between the baby and the mother. Also a mother without extra aid doesn't hand over at a certain hour or when she desperately needs it.

The basic care involves the sleeping, the feeding, the cooking, the bathing, the (re)dressing, the entertainment, the emotional wellbeing, the stimulation, the relaxation, the parenting and the education of baby and yourself. I'm mentioning "the" because it is not something you can ever skip on or be flexible about. They need to be done, constantly, in a constant flow throughout the day and the night. In the meantime you should also be dressed, energized, fed, educated and as your messing up the household, you will spend more time and energy on cleaning up your mess and reorganizing your house.
You'll also want to relax the mind on social media and setup a business. Setup a business? I mean that sarcastically, but it is the truth. Every mother also wants a career and often she'll think of something that is more "she" as a mother and which will give her the chance to quit her job and work from home or at least be flexible with her schedule. For me it was writing a book and moving houses, but for others it involves clients, products, handcrafting, studying or pursuit of a new career. Your new activity as a stay at home mom (sahm), might be to attend a lot of play groups and even organize them yourself. Is it physically possible to do all this besides the overwhelming and daunting tasks of the sahm? It is different for each person, couple, home, situation, although one thing is sure; each SAHM is not only overwhelmed with the actual tasks of the job but also by

herself. She is confronted with her inner world, her inner obstacles, her new challenges, her loneliness, her devalue, her sanity, her aspirations, her inflexibility and the list goes on. We will get more into that matter later on in the book.

Creche: can't give you a right or wrong answer. I think it's a huge dilemma and some parents find a better balance within themselves than others or are more convinced about what they want for themselves: which sacrifices they are willing to make for themselves or for their baby. Each parent and each baby and each life are different in a way, so its not a copy paste situation, even between your own children.

In the nursery baby's main activity is to be on its own, instead of interacting his thoughts and feelings with his conscious mom or dad. The caretaker and even other family members cannot replace the mom or dad. Here we might find a main difference between a parent and a conscious parent: a conscious mom or dad will want to interact on the thoughts, feelings and behavior of their baby and the guidance and development of such for the best will, the inner and outer wellness, of the developing child and the "future adult". If you cannot provide these hours or the majority of these hours until 6-7 months of age, you might not be conscious about the wellbeing and outmost importance for their inner and outer wellbeing. This provides as a warning that if possible, you can save your salaries to provide this time away from the job or seek another solution. Mine was to quit the job, have them resign me, sell the house and move to a cheaper apartment. Another possibility would have been to take a sick leave or an extended maternity or paternity which normally parents in Belgium would take up to age twelve.

To cut through the chase, there is also the possibility to BYOB, bring your own baby, to work that is. If you have a clinic, shop, an office or you are the boss, this might very well work for you. Of course it needs adjustments and provides challenges, but so does staying at home.

What is the difference between home and a nursery?
In the nursery baby's main activity is too be on its own, with his own thoughts and feelings in a group setting: there are other babies and older children. The babies usually are crying from periods at time and the toddlers will be running and making noise. Some nurseries do not provide structured activities for the toddlers. Until the baby can crawl, they will sit on a chair for hours in a row or have tummy time for an extended period. Personally I don't think that is attractive at all.
Breastfeeding, bonding, communication, attachment, connection and learning from mommy (or daddy) is not an option. On a mental level, baby is learning about a school setting during these hours and not on the experience of family, family members, close relationships, body development, mind control and such unconscious conditions. There is no research on this specific subject, it's solely an observation of the hours spent 'at school' v.s. 'with mom or other family'. A balance between both worlds can be more ideal. It also depends on type of character your baby has which determines if your baby thrives in a school setting and from what month in the Diamond year or from what month be-

yond the first year. Use that as an indicator when your baby (and you) are thriving with a nursery + home combination.

Integrated family time
If we don't invest family time consciously or unconsciously either during the day, in the evening or in the weekends during baby's first and second year, than automatically and logically 'family experience' cannot be an integrate experience within the conscious or subconscious of the baby. The main relationship of a baby in the first year is either with mom or another (main) caretaker, but there needs to be one reliable one. Baby cannot connect with all caretakers equally. If there is not a main caretaker, baby will have a sense of dis-belonging to this world, perhaps 'losing oneself', a trust issue or a bonding issue. If this is what we learn and are taught about life, than why would that necessarily change later on and as an adult? Perhaps the parents can make an effort to reverse the effect in the brain and subconscious of the baby in year 2,3,4 but it will need some dedication and compensation. Again, there is no official research done as far as I know and in this book we assume, from a logic point of view, that the first year of baby out of the womb is the first introduction and the base of how life is experienced. The first year is the primal year of baby's growth, it is memorized within the cells, brain structure, subconscious as well as conscious behavior of the child as he grows up. When the baby starts to walk, we can assume that the first year of his life has been integrated and is now put to practice.

Relationships and their foundations
Relationships of a tot and toddler are either with mom or with another main caretaker up to four years old. So if it is not you; than who is the main caretaker? And again: does baby get the same things and same quality from the other caretaker? Being possibly breastfed and growth through physical closeness with the mother is invaluable. How do you see the world if you were to look through baby's eyes? What would become your inward perspective on the world an life?
We can't always judge from the outside what is going on from the inside. The same concept applies to adults. We don't all have the same filter to receive life and perceive it. Our personalities, experience and consciousness make life what it is for us personally. No matter what we do or don't do in life, both for children and adults it's the inside that we are forming, shaping, cultivating. Children just have much more of a clean slate and are a bigger challenge as they grow up. It's up to you as a parent to judge and see what this means to you and ultimately your baby's first year. What are you going to do and not do in order to shape your baby's inner world? As well, the years to come as they come. The first year cannot be repeated though and that is something I wish to stress out in favour of your baby and for you as an adult to have a maximum sense of balance and wellbeing.

Bonding is communication
Besides breastfeeding the other main task of baby is learning to bond and communicate, how do you see this process unfolding if you are not there most of the time? Learning to

bond and learning to communicate is both an internal and external process. When baby (or adult) communicate or try to communicate they send out a messages from one inner world to another inner world. Communication can be a combination of words, emotions, feelings, body expressions and sounds from the inside world. The response (or no response) that is given from 'the outside world' is significant to the response that will be felt on the inside world. We call this conditioning.

Conditioning is the inner dialogue we have with ourselves, between ourselves and with the outside world. But in reality there is no outside world. We attach thoughts, feeling and emotions to the outside world, even to people, so in fact we are only communicating with ourselves. This conditioning stays with us for a life time and is always active, we don't suddenly lose or gain it as adults. It just becomes a stronger conditioning over the years. There is a constant inner dialogue that takes place between you as a grown up person and your small inner child. We can almost imagine there is no actual adult, there is only the inner child up to an age of seven years old disguised in the body suit of an adult. The adult behaves in a certain way, which is conditioned by society, but on the inside there is the seven year old. The inner child being you with the full recording of your childhood up to seven years of age. After that, it does not matter much what we get or don't get out of life, because we live in unconsciousness until we hit the age of 21 and again at 28 and probably every 7 years thereafter we get a rude wake up call. The subconscious does not and never does stop recording your life as it unfolds before your eyes. It's exactly like a tape recorder or a videocamera constantly 'on'.

How does this relate to growing up in a creche or school? When your baby is in a day care, the baby will have the (unconscious) recording of 'being at school' from the age of six weeks. It's as simple as that. The subconscious cannot differentiate between different possible experiences or states of being or options which perhaps start at the age of 21 or 28 or even later on. The younger subconscious has only one option: the one it is presented. It simply records whatever is given from the outside as well from the reflections on the inside.

Twinkle, Twinkle, Little Star... Where are you?

Sleeping at the nursery is not exactly ideal, especially if the nursery didn't take care of a specialised room where the babies will sleep or if they disturb one another too much. There is hardly a quiet setting: the toddlers are being active and other babies might be crying non-stop. How would you enjoy these settings for your quiet time and sleep? Ideally, I imagine a nursery for small babies with soft colors and quiet sounds and a full-on caretaker, distanced from the other children in the creche. The baby's day should be focused only on sleep, drinking milk, hygiene routines and playful moments, until they start solids and sitting up. And on the occasion, only in those rare moments of playful cycles the babies are taken to the play corner or stimulated in a certain skill. Breastfeeding is near to impossible if your baby goes to the creche.

If your baby didn't get to experience the bonding phase or relations with mommy and other family members, surely your child will encounter the experience more and more consciously at a different age. There will be celebrations, maybe early on at play dates or with the extended family.

Your child will absorb, not from a primal development in the first year's brain development, but from his more conscious 'mind' in a later stage. He will learn, some way or another, what it means to be in a relation with close ones. There is no wrong or right here. I'm only making an observation. And without extensive research there is no true or false. We don't need to wait on science for making personal choices and constructing our children and family life. I'm merely offering you here the possibility and insights through conscious observation and a bit of literature that the development of the brain, the inner dialogue (conditioning) and the subconscious can be enriched in the primal phase and that it does serve for a life time.

Bonding and becoming whole again
In the nursery there is an overstimulation of group and society's socialization with the other group members at the creche, but there is an under stimulation of being with mom, dad or other family members. The four walls are the limits of baby's world and experience. This is contrary to the typical observation that the creche is to socialize the baby and that if this is skipped you'll have an unsocial baby. There is a phase for everything and socializing with the outside world is something for month 6 or 7 until month 12. Being social has nothing to do with the amount of hours spent with colleagues, it has everything to do with how the

baby is bonded and what it is taught about relationships and especially communication. Communication including our own inner dialogue, brought forth by conditioning as mentioned earlier, is the base of all relationships.

Being social comes from an inner confidence. When there is inner confidence, this can followed by a solid connectedness and experience in the outside world. We can be surrounded with 1000's of fans and still feel lonely and isolated. How come? Ask the stars from the music and the screens how lonely they have felt at times. The stay-at-home baby can experience the world and relations through the mother and their experiences together not only in the home, but at the meet-ups, at the stores, the parks, family gatherings, doing the groceries, on the streets, at the swimming pool, at coffee mornings, play groups and during extended holidays… Daily tasks become an integral experience for baby and for mommy to learn about and bond with her baby. She transmits her inner confidence an the bond with humanity is established. Baby is welcomed in this world. A world of materialism, barriers, conflicts and separation. Only to learn again what it is to be 'whole again', this time through the flesh.

In the nursery, they are however structured, hygienic and incredible in doing THE job. But this is a superficial and a clinical approach to raising a baby. As a mother, you are given less of a chance to go through the personal growth of yourself and the bond with your child. The nursery also means there is no or less bathing, redressing, carrying and so on. At home you have these tasks which make the days more intense opposed the professional's job. In the nursery there is less availability and there is a group structure or social pressure which the baby usually will adapt to. With that structure and no attention from mommy, it could also help your baby to sleep better. Baby adapts, yes. Why would he not? Wouldn't you adapt to a situation if you were not given another option? Adaptation is a survival mechanism. Again, there is no right or wrong. All solutions have advantages and disadvantages for either you or your baby. You are the only judge to tell if your child is happy and if you are being happy with the choices that you can and cannot make. The dilemma will probably remain and is common to parents, but at least you should feel that you had a 50% choice.

On the outlook for your tribe

A social network can be built offline as well online. Your online community, like a Facebook group, forums or instagram followers can give you direct or indirect support and answers your questions if needed. You are reaching out to a bigger group of people and like-minded. Your offline network will be able to help you out and share experiences more directly and from a close surroundings, which will make you less lonely in the process. We've all been there.

My husband and I are an expatriated couple living in a country without any family member. Most family members live in neighboring countries and others live on 3000+ miles by flight. In a short to chase, practical sense this means I'm lacking free and trusted babysitters and never get a break.

Even if you are now limited to go out on dates with your partner, due to the lack of babysitting, there are still possibilities for you to go out and hit a party. You can split up.

There is a weekly Guys'- and Girls'- night out. Not necessarily with a bigger group of girls or guys, it could be with a single friend. The other options you can think of:

- Home dinners, parties or movie nights at your place
- Home dinners, parties or movie nights at a friend's place
- Dress up parties, with any random theme that you think of at home
- Seasonal traditions, what better time than starting your family traditions now
- Baby and mom get-togethers
- Baby and parents get-togethers in the weekend, maybe a picnic in the park or a very child friendly restaurant. Some cities have family restaurants, other than fast-food and I've even been at a restaurant with their own daycare

These parties where baby can (partly) take part and then go to sleep, is not only good for you to party and socialize, it's also good for your baby to socialize. When they socialize with adults these adults will become like aunts and uncles on a more individual level as they get to know your baby. They don't see just a 'baby', they see a personality and either someone they respect or someone to play with. Your baby will feel indirectly supported as an individual and part of a 'tribe', even later on, knowing that him and his parents have and had support from friends, neighbors, framily, etc.

When you are meeting with those supportive adults and other babies, you can keep a list of names and pictures for your baby to connect back to when he's grown up. Maybe he will recontact these individuals as they have shared important moments of their history.

Family support or strain?
Have you relied on you husband before? Perhaps during a time of illness or financial lack? How was he? Was he supportive? Is he already tired of doing it again? How is your family relating to you during your pregnancy? Were there any hardships before being married or pregnant? It does not need to be a rule of thumb, although this is what to expect while expecting. Patterns can change, but they are not in favor to change, as they have been patterns for years. So be vigilant with your birth plans and postpartum plan in the first days, weeks and months. Be prepared to switch plans swiftly if things are not working out in the best of your favor or to best circumstances with family members.
One of my friends had a great experience with her mother as a grandmother, although she had a terribly toxic relationship as mother - daughter. Her mother was apparently very comfortable as a grandmother and had no issue of her own daughter being a mother.

True motivations and passion pull in life
Perfect chance to get in touch with your true motivations. What theme or problem in this world makes you tick. What do you think about most? What is it that you are good at? What is it that you actually have always been doing? What is it that you recognize yourself for or others recognize in you? We can call this passion, the passion that lives in our bodies, minds and souls. It could literally be anything.

Little things can lead to big things. Maybe you'll start a crafty thing which you made for you baby / child. Maybe you will make some sort of "come back" from an earlier job or career. Maybe you will feel the "now or never" of setting up a business of your own or go back to study for new certificates. I remember, at one time, I developed educational activity boxes with my ex-boyfriend for the regular school system. Now I'm back with passion for informing and educating adults and children on their personal skills and development.

Play Mate

We find online connection through the loss of connection. This is not only the phenomena of the children in a tech-age; it is the parents that live in the tech-age. Instead of the absent, narcotic or obsessed parent, we find the internet freak has replaced the parent. The child naturally finds its way to the internet and social media which broadens its horizons by the day. As a parent, we are the helper and the play mate of our tech-obsessed child and selves. We need to balance the act throughout the day and compensate between being human and being online.

The relation between Attachment and Addiction

The first thing and perhaps only thing that the parents have to be aware of is attachment, From the moment the woman is pregnant to the daily routine and struggles of childhood, tweens, teenage and young adulthood. It is all about attachment. Every problem comes forth of a lack of attachment, including all sorts of addictions. Separation instead of bonding is a roadway to hell. To be aware of attachment is the essential quality in attachment parenting and conscious parenting. How to acknowledge attachment if you were not attached to yourself, life and your loved ones? How to make yourself, the feminine and the mom happy and functional? We need to practice and continue practicing self-love which starts with self-care.

CHART

What is Self-Care?

Nutrition for you! Juices, smoothies, bowls, shakes! And a glass of alcohol or a big fat cake once a while to kill the nerves and the healthy lifestyle.

Natural aroma's on your skin and in the diffuser, on your clothing, on your sheets

Music for you in the room and through head phones!

Touch for you! Cuddle, massage, dates with your partner and more. Chiropractor (you and baby)

Comfort at your social worker or psychologist, parent support groups, the gym and out of the house on your own

Safety from help around you helping you out with household, cleaning, groceries, cooking, baby sitting and driving around. You are in it together.

Security are emotions related to bonding, space and attachment to life and the world. Seeking security is related to authority, boundaries and guidance which are now given by yourself by self-parenting and re-parenting.

Your looks matter! When you look good, you feel good. You will need an extra budget and time to keep up with those rocking looks and a stash of beauty products and accessories that make that quick fix.

The MOM Job and Sleepception

Now that we spoke about the importance for your baby physical growth, let's talk about the importance for you to have recognition for the job you are doing.

1. The MOM job comes with responsibilities and tasks.
2. The MOM job comes without hours, it is 24/7.

Meaning, these hours are 24 hours per day, 7 days per week, no- breaks, weekends, holidays or switch of profession or employer.
Yes, baby is a cruel boss. On top of all that, you will have a guarantee of chronic lack of sleep (sleep deprivation). Sleep has become what I call "sleepception"; the concept of sleep as in there might have been sleep or their might not have been any hour of sleep. Sleep deprivation can and does cause a series of discomfort, frustrations, burn-out and disease. Sleep deprivation is common to all working and worried people, especially high performing and overworked people. The MOM job is both and all, to the next level, it is in my eyes qualified as a high performance job. Although it is not recognized as one by government, corporations, society or self. Stress related issues and total burnouts have never been more common than this age and time, that includes moms.

In fact, this job is for the next x years to come, until baby has phased out of childhood into adulthood. And even in adulthood we can lose our sleep over the worries and problems of our child.

Life is not meant to be hard work. Nature looks for the road
of least resistance. Look at how electricity or water flows
through a materialised object. And we are exactly that: water
and electricity. It's our life intention and destiny. But maybe
because we were the fighter amongst all those sperm cells,
we believe in survival of the fittest when it comes to our life's
management. We need to struggle, we think.

Determination and decisions alone is not enough, we think.
Somehow it doesn't work in making us a
happier, more fulfilling human being. We need to unlearn
what we have learned. That's why it's worth searching for the
other, right path that will lead to joy not merely as a
happiness goal, but as a state of being.

The MOM Job can be qualified a high performance job. - Andromeda L.C.

The hours that you, as a parent, wish to take off from your job means that another qualified person will take over your job for those amount of hours, even minutes of the day or night.

A baby / child cannot be left unattended for even the amount of one minute. It is in fact the kind of boss that is on top of your shoulders - all of the time, all of the time. Yes, he or she is cruel. For the parent, only a physical separation could truly ease the body and mind. As long as they are awake, we worry about them and of course tend to their every need. They are very needy of things, us and all kinds of attention.

So even if you are not ON the job clocking your minutes, someone else will be doing it for you and you will most likely be depending on good will or you are paying for a professional. These qualified people are: creche, school, after school daycare or activities, grandparents, other family members, neighbors, friends, babysitters or nannies, other moms and of course your partner, the other parent.

But how come you are not being paid for this job?
Because they are your children. You know how they say you are borrowing your children? Particularly from God. Even if you don't believe in God or Consciousness or - you name it -, something inside your body has created this magnificent human and is keeping it "Alive and Kicking" outside of your body. In some sense: they are not yours. They will grow up believing that 'they are their own' anyway. You will need to have the humongous sense that they are your responsibility in close cooperation with the community around you. Imagine a nursery or school does not feel the responsibility? What kind of school would that be? Would you drop your child at such a school? Probably not. So they say, God chose you to borrow (t)his particular child. Like a school, with full trust.

Now comes the Job Description:

Responsibilities & Tasks of The MOM Job
- Keep the child safe every second and minute of the day and night by your own profession or by a qualified person that you have carefully selected that can take over all of your responsibilities and tasks.
- Keep the working environment healthy, clean and pleasant. Add or distract any furniture, accessories or ambiance and energy for the right settings for the boss (the child) and you (ass well as other colleagues that might be sharing your space).
- Keep the child in good health when it's tending to go into a bad health or habit (this responsibility will not stop far into adulthood).
- Teach the child basic human survival skills and about it's own body.
- Teach the child basic social skills and behavior (this responsibility will continue into adulthood).
- Keep a daily hygiene of the child: bathing, showering hair, brushing the hair, cleaning nails, cleaning the nose, cleaning the ears, etc.
- Dress the child appropriately to weather conditions and with some sense of fashion.
- Teach the child to brush it's teeth independently and to do this on a daily routine (up to 3 times per day).
- As child is not capable of going to the toilets, change the diaper as many times and as soon as possible. Can be a minimum of 5 times per day.
- Educate the child about literature, animal world, plant world, mechanics etc.
- Feed the child the required dose of foods and nutrition preferably the first months with your breasts,

later on with bottles and than with healthy solids (in the first half year to year feeding is a guarantee of every 2,5-6 hours, day and night. The proceeding years until adulthood this task will not stop).
- Take intensive care and find the correct healing solutions for the child when he is at discomfort or disease, being ill (guaranteed in the first years)
- Wake up and take intensive care when the child is awake or in discomfort at night (guaranteed in the first years).
- Entertain the child so he doesn't get bored. Guide the child while doing things that he/she likes to do in that moment or that particular day.
- Take care of a healthy brain development from the start and do not cause any type of addictions earlier or later on (example: excessive electronics like tv, smartphone, tablet, pc, gaming etc).
- Discipline the child so you can have a smooth cooperation and for a pleasant cowering existence with other colleagues and associates.
- Potty train poo and pee during day and night for the first 3+ years.
- Keep yourself in good health by investing in yourself during the hours on the job, as the job does not include free-time. There will not be sufficient time, neither mornings or nights, to take much care of your own hygiene, appearance or dress up (sorry for that).
- Work on your internal self (preferably on a 2 daily basis), your relationships, your self- and world image and your company department in order to

evolve, smooth out any obstacles and constructively build on future plans of the company.
- Make yourself some money so you can sense a value for your existence, have semi-independency or have independency whilst doing this job.
- Money can be made when the boss is in training outside of the office (preferably not in the first probation year) into When the boss is in training hours or if you decide to outsource your job.
- Your office will be in your home, cafe's, playrooms, parcs, shops. Whilst you are in the office, we expect you to take care of the environment as mentioned previously and serve to the colleagues that share the office with you as you are the most qualified senior. This includes tasks as: dishes in/out, groceries, meal preparations 1-3 times p/day, cleaning daily hazards and stains, arrangements, vacuuming, cleaning the fridge, taking out garbage, cleaning the windows, change bed sheets, take care of pets and plants. You have the possibility to delegate these tasks, but be aware that your senior position does not impress your other colleagues and we cannot (at all) guarantee a daily, weekly or monthly cooperation.
- Doing groceries for you, your child and other colleagues in the company.
- Be an every day and long term example to your child in order to set the example for a healthy society, an internally happy person and an contributor to his and other lives. Be an inspiration for the good, not the bad.
- Love this child.

Special Note
This is an unpaid job with no means of salary or compensation - actually it will cost you a whole lot of money as you are paying the life of this person. He or she needs rent of a bigger place to stay, extra bills, edutainment, special needs and a lot of supplies and demands. Once you started, you cannot quit and you do not want to quit.

As you tend to be involved in this job in the future you might have a second or third "boss baby" to attend to with the same responsibilities and tasks. We will not be able to hire an assistant for neither you nor your new boss, as you are the only qualified person for this boss and considering the lack of financial means this usually is not a possibility.

Note from your Boss
In future conditions we hope to have a company growth and better financial means in order to compensate for a job well done. We are also sorry to mention that you will not be trained for the job, neither will you have further training as these will be minutes lost attending your child or catching up on lack of sleep. If you can still manage to pursue any training, money accumulation or business development, whilst keeping up the responsibilities and tasks (or somehow outsourcing some tasks) than we encourage you to do so, as this job, contrary to the kind of intelligence that is required and the high standards that we seek after, the job might or will become dull quickly due to the character of the boss and the lack of "you-time".

Personally, we think me-time (or "you" time) is overrated for this kind of job as you have chosen to entirely devote yourself voluntarily, not only to the job, but to the boss (or two or three) and his/her existence. We do encourage you to become a better person and a better performer. No need to say that you will be evaluated, more than once per year and by more than several significant others as well as the mainstream on your overall performance as well as school, society and community. All that criticism is positive feedback that we expect you to take seriously. Your boss(es) will also be evaluating you on a regular basis and giving you the necessary feedback.

Keeping the engine running

As you become sensitive to which energy you are using (male, female, physical, mental, emotional, spiritual) in a certain moment, your next step is to become sensitive to how and when to use them. If one is depleted, than move on to another by doing an activity that suits that energy bucket. You will have the chance to feel re-energized!

You as a parents need to alternate between the two parents; the child needs both and needs both male and female energy to be with them on a daily or weekly basis.

Male energy is RED; doing, re-active, active, goal oriented and achieving, oriented around tasks, factual.

Female energy is PINK; being, receptive as well as responsive, not centered around tasks, rather it takes all the time it needs for fruition, imaginative.

Play with these colors in your mind and in your wardrobe, accessories, agenda or household. Alternate between these two energies to have enough energy management throughout the day. Also consider that you have three types of energy buckets to deplete and refill: physical, emotional, mental, spiritual.

If you have emptied a bucket and continue the activity, you are driving on a burn out. A phone call with a friend or family member can recharge your emotional bucket and give you a renewed energy as well to recharge your day. A rest of the eyes using your spiritual energy to be recharged can refill your physical and mental buckets. A few minutes or some hours in nature or doing something crafty can refill your buckets on many levels, in order to refresh and recharge for the next week. The list goes on. It's for you to become more aware about and to play with, without feeling guilty. It is important for us humans and our children of modern age to understand flow, play and energy in order to be more human and less robotic (and less online). So when you are tired, ask yourself, what am I tired of? And than how can I recharge one or two of my buckets?

4 Daddy Depression and Anger Management

them too

The first baby is a big change and chance to accelerate your life as an individual as well as a couple. Accepting the change (and chance) is the biggest challenge for the individual and the couple. Living up to the family you have created is the key to life time happiness.

For the daddy, one of the main worries on his mind is his fear of the unknown and the cost of living. These come forth from a sense of responsibility, but this sense of responsibility can be overwhelming causing the man to flee to the inside of himself or to the outside of the home.

I wish to create this awareness that daddies are as much affected as mothers are affected by her pregnancy and motherhood. It is somehow unfair to say that the father does not get affected because the mother has carried out the pregnancy, the breastfeeding and most of the care-taking. A father is as much pregnant and as much on board of fatherhood. We just don't see it on a physical level or in the particular lifestyle. It's not expressed and talked about as much as the pregnancy of a woman and the arrival of the new baby. But why not? Why are the dads not speaking as much or spoken about as much? I didn't know one expectant dad that was not either very excited to have the pregnancy of the baby or was simply very scared of the new, awaited arrival.

These men spoke about it and the majority of dads are with their wives and families, contrary to their possibility of living separately form them. I even believe that the majority of divorced dads are the most affected by the separation in case of separation, more so than the women. So where is the father in this picture of pregnancy and baby's arrival? Which support does he get? Where does he get the attention from the spot light, the joy of celebration at a baby shower and the concern for his overall health? And still, they are patiently by our side, the female, despite all the "nagging" and changes in their household.

What can a father do in the first weeks, months, year and years to come:

- Have a sense of responsibility

- Have a sense of fatherhood
- Build onward on the family unit
- Creating contact with his baby
- Creating affection for his wife and family
- Waking up at night
- Changing diapers
- Preparing and giving a bottle
- Have baby while mom goes for me-time
- Logistics and give rides
- Cook
- Cuddle and rough play
- Watch a baby cartoon or movie together
- Nap together
- Carry around in baby sling
- Play live music or songs with baby
- Dad can take a bath with Baby
- Set up all the new gadgets and technology in the home
- Take a stroll with baby in the stroller
- Go to the park or play ground, meet other dads
- Do playdates with other parents

- Picnic with baby and friends (not too many beers! in order to keep attention with baby)
- Do whatever daddies do best with their children!

Dad can set up comfy nursing spots around the house and make sure Mama eats well. It doesn't sound like a glamorous, bonding job; but supporting Mom to support Baby is a tremendous and touching gift! If she is not nourished well, she can't nourish Baby. The woman's male energy can be exerted with a freelance job or studying on the laptop or whilst outside of the home.

The imbalance of Patriarch and Matriarch

If males are grown and intertwined with a form of machoism, which is present in some cultures more than others, perhaps the majority of (sub)cultures, that's another challenge for the father to adapt to an age and expectations of equality that have become far less patriarch. Machoism can be: I don't change diapers, I don't push the stroller, I don't hold babies. Something they best get rid of by the time they have the actual baby! And still, who is helping these dads breaking the taboo and norm? A child needs both parents and the partners need to depend on each other for help which is both practical and emotional. Fortunately, almost all men I have met and seen in western, Arab and Latin cultures were happy to fully participate in their baby's growth and care. On a side note: the Arab (and Lebanese) culture is very much involved with their babies and children, in contrary to popular belief. In case the dad is half or not involved, which surely, I've also seen and experienced in men from Western and Arab culture, the dad can become partly absent and the woman can become partly bitter. Also, in a world of freedom for individuality and equality, we are all seeking for our individual lives to be lived up to potential and fulfilling, not solely to work for money or for the household. So the individual life of the mother, just like the father, includes certain type of career or other work and priorities, only one of them being motherhood.

Fatherhood will in turn bring out the female energy within the man, which is a very healthy balance of the yin and yang energy we all possess. His female side will nurture in a way he has been perhaps unfamiliar with, at least in the context of having a family, it becomes very fulfilling and nurturing for his soul and self-esteem as he is becoming a more whole person. It also creates extra empathy for the role of the mother and the effort she does in her many, long and dedicated hours carrying the weight of the children on her responsibility. Men are empathic naturally, they usually are not given this chance through our matriarch system. We tend to believe it is the Patriarch that causes our men to be out of sync with their feminine energy: the receiving, the calm, the quiet, the sensing, the interconnecting, the breath, the love. When in reality it was their mothers that have withheld them from growing into a whole human being. The mothers have withheld them from exposing or nurturing their feminine energy because they were brought up either too manly in our society or from a broken mother, whose female side was not nurtured. So both men and women are missing the feminine, the Ying energy, in their daily lives. But it lives within us. And it is hurting. This is what true feminism is about: the balance of the sexual energies within us. As well as the becoming of equal, mutually respected individuals. And by being only half our energy, our yang, a man will be half a man and a woman will be half a woman.

A full grown human is comprised of both yang and Ying, male and female energy. As is the adult woman when she regains and steps into her female energy. Women have become and learnt to be men in our societies. Men have a stronger sense of the female or feminine, but they feel like they cannot give this enough space in their inner world and their lives. It can form a source of judgement, abandonment, exclusion. It is said: "Men don't cry and they don't have a heart". Unfortunately our modern societies are suffering from the lack of Motherly Love. The Ancient cultures, native cultures, are not as much affected by this imbalance. Perhaps it was the heavy migrations, agriculture and industrialization that contributed to the imbalance. I believe the Roman culture, which the Western culture is built upon, adored both male and female energy in both males and females. Both were gods, both were cultivated, both were appreciated. A men could have been very elegant and a woman could have been very bold. The mother figure, as head of a matriarch, was more easily accepted as they are within native cultures. Women are wise women, the wise elderly, the medicine woman, the enchantress, the wild woman, the crone, the council, the wife of, the warrior princess and so on. Whilst nowadays, we are denigrating women in our thoughts and mainstream culture wether they are a career "bitch" or a SAHM "stay at home mom" which both by title are inclined to be insults. It is a complex world with total lack of respect and be aware; not by lack of respect from men per se, but lack of respect from women. Women are designing the advertisements and shaping the catwalk models as much as men are. Don't tell me there are no women in advertisement and they cant put a man behind the stove, the dishes and the laundry. And they too buy soap and know sometimes better than women how to clean stains, spots and such. I know my husband knows much better than me and my European male friend does all the laundry of the baby. The Arab from The Gulf wear thobes and are an expert keeping their white cotton extremely fresh throughout the day by a full set of techniques of washing a possible stain on the go. They also don't mind at all to push the baby trolly, hold the baby or assist their small children. They actually enjoy it.

Disrespecting our Mothers

Every man was born out of a woman and if he lacks respect for his mother, it might have been that as he was growing into manhood, into young adulthood, he was overpowered, controlled or had another individual confrontation with his mother. As long as the mother is not whole herself and comes from a place of lack, she is likely to inflict damage to her son - especially a son as her counter-self. The girls can outgrow their pain for not being seen and not being empowered, a man will remain caged forever. I believe so. These chains need a cultural breakthrough. I feel like this is still uncommon grounds and perhaps the real feminism rising: women need to become whole, so men will be allowed to have their feminine counter self through their motherly love and respect. They can become better men and a better society, alongside the women.

Equality in partnership

In order for the definition of "dad" to be one of an equal partner in the act of child-care, fathers must be active participants from day one. This early bonding sets the stage for a positive relationship in later years, and helps the family build a strong and equal foundation for child-rearing. This is easier said than done and is most successful if the father naturally has the right attitude towards children, family and pregnancy from his own upbringing or education. If he has been trained and accustomed before the birth event of serving and utilizing his softer-male side, he is miles ahead. Same goes for the tough women. It is a wild ride if you will wait on the dad becoming a dad by himself. He needs the right support, just like the pregnant or postpartum woman usually needs and might get her support.

With strong desire, motivation, and support, fathers can be involved (and knowledgeable) in everything from buying baby formula to finding the right nanny and nurturing the parent-caregiver relationship. Obstacles are a natural part of any significant shift in societal perceptions — but fathers shouldn't let outdated expectations or views affect how they care for their families, because the 21st century dad is well on his way to being accepted as an equal partner in caring for his family beyond the role of the breadwinner."

Daddy Depression exists and it is as real as PSTD (post stress traumatic disorder) of mothers.

- Unknown

Men get depressed too

Men too get depressed after the baby arrives. Either they have the postpartum depression or they are getting depressed because of your situation and depression. Learn to recognize the symptoms, so you can both get help, which in any case, you should both have help to deal with your very normal, every day kind of situation. All parents go through these phases, for some it is just much and much worse than for others. I also think this depression can come and go with phases depending on how the household is run, how their job is doing, how well they have eaten or if they have partnered recently. Here are some example thoughts which you might recognize as your own:

"I was hoping to find a happy home"

"Where is the dinner"

"Where is the romance"

"The house is dark and gloomy"

"My wife is crying all the time"

"The baby is crying a lot"

"There is a complete mess everywhere"

Going back to "normal" does not exist

You are not alone. Many new and current parents go through this awfully depressing phase and wish it would be "normal" again. Or normal with a baby. But, it never seems to become normal. You can have a happy time, only if you are both very understanding and soft in your approach. A baby involves more work than one, two or even three persons can handle! Many modern day families wish they could afford a nanny, yet the ones that have a nanny see a complexity of the parental role and couple's guilt and blame.

The mother's body is in a state of physical, emotional, mental shock after the birth and with the continuous care for the baby. Both lives had a big impact, a big hit, and you have yet to realize it. It will get better. You will grow to be a family. You will grow to be happy. One day. You will grow to be parents. You will take back a life of your own. It needs dedication, a whole lot of patience and mutual understanding.

What is postpartum depression or postpartum anxiety about?

Postpartum depression or anxiety is a biochemical disorder. I believe it can happen, or will happen, to both the woman and the man. Certainly, the depression will happen to the woman and the anxiety might come harder for the man. When the brain's chemistry returns to normal, the wife and mother will feel like herself again. When the household is more stabilized, the woman is back on her feet and the baby has grown out of his first year, the man too will find more peace. This can happen around month 6-8, but it is still in a fragile state and will stabilize more after the first birthday. It is the partner's role to support the mother and wife as this is happening and to ask what she needs at any given moment just to get through the days, weeks and year. She will know and she should feel secure enough to tell you. It's no-one's fault that this is happening and she cannot fix it easily at all. This is part of becoming a stronger couple and growing into the family. We are not adventures, romantic partners anymore, the family demands an attitude of serving and self sacrifice. Let the mother sleep as much as possible, put friendly or professional help on a schedule, order food to the house, get a cleaning lady and lower your expectations of the wife, girlfriend and mother. In this crucial period, you are partners and there are many responsibilities to keep the train running. You will learn to be partners for the rest of your life if you survive this. Don't judge, don't criticize and don't compare. This is not the time to get fussy about details or even the bigger picture. Not all tasks can be done in life or around the house, survival is the next standard. If everyone is in safety and in health, it is the biggest achievement of all! If you made any other progressions, that is a great bonus.

Comparison kills

If the partner is not considerate or already suffering from postnatal depression himself, you may be a contributor or source of depression by making severe or continuous mistakes. The common things that husbands do is comparing his wife to other women. This is extremely confusing and hurtful to the wife's sense of self-esteem and self-worth. Why has becoming a mother, become a big issue in the marriage? Of course she is not the first to give birth or to have a baby, but it is the first time for her! No, she does not have 2,3, 7 or 12 children but neither do you, right? You go to work every day, but your salary didn't double it's size because you have a child now, did it? The mother didn't inherit all the skills, experience, energy and recipes from your grandmother while giving birth.

Cry your heart out

Crying after the experience of birth and after sleepless nights and desperation over the baby is all the reason to cry. As a woman, we've lost so much and gained so much, all in once and we have no good support network to catch all the falling pieces. Crying is the least we can do. As a partner we can put our arms around our partner and give comfort and tell them it will be alright with time. Looking for practical solutions together to organize your life, like brining clothing to the dry cleaning and pre-ordering (frozen) dishes or recipe boxes, will make the situation less depressing and lonely. Once you know you are both working on the practical organization and working on it together, you are planning your family's ease and happiness. Besides, you don't know what goes on behind closed doors of the people that you know and don't know. Comparison is a killer.

Men's anger and outrage

Getting angry from a feeling of insecurity is not a conscious decision, especially if you cannot make up for it right away. A men's anger will express itself through humiliation and threats, which both are extremely damaging to the marriage and the foundation of friendship and trust (which might have not been there in the first place). You might end up divorcing for this exact reason. And it's not a little reason. I wouldn't be surprised if new mothers, even with the second or third baby, get physically beaten just because of being a new mother (again) and being in the weak, vulnerable position. If I've met you, I wanted to forget about you. Poor parents. This is what you suffer in the desperation of your own hurt Inner Child, your anger and your despair with a child in your midst.

The responsibility and breadwinner legacy

It's very frustrating to new fathers to see and deal with this new situation. They feel as they've lost their wife, their anchor. They lost their girlfriend and they wonder why they are even with this woman. At the same time, they feel an enormous sense of responsibility as a caretaker of finance and security. Both towards the wife and the child(ren). This sense of responsibility is not always logic or rationalized. It seems to come through the DNA. The best case for both partners is to talk openly and honestly about all the burdens. Everything is new and nothing will come as a big surprise when you can talk about the question marks. It will come as a bigger surprise when we, especially women, are confronted with anger, resentment, criticism, denigration and threats.

Working longer hours or not coming home at all are even more lame for a man to turn into a habit, because you still have a longterm responsibility towards the baby and it's main caretaker. If you are going to stay out to breath, just tell her so and give her that same opportunity! Your wife is usually not permanently ill or handicapped after birth, she just needs to recover, to have her alone time, to see friends without her baby and to do normal adult stuff. The situation is very hard on you, because all of a sudden you have not a sick, but an ill partner. And you have a baby and you have yourself to deal with. It's a lot. The thing that can help you is to realize:

1. She is not permanently ill and she's not sick (usually), she is overworked with her baby and her own body.

2. You can give her all the relief! Let her take her rest, feed her tummy and let her off the hook so she can go out of the home.

A joint venture

Making your wife's health and therefore the well-being of your family your number one priority is the best thing you can do as a husband. Your wife will carry the rest of the load and find her way towards the best way for your family and "how things can be done". She will probably want to do this as a team and you will have your important contribution to the family, not only financially but also with your intelligence and practical input. A house, family and well-being are a joint venture. They are not and have never been only on the shoulders of a woman. It's wrong to think that men in a traditional role or of the earlier decades were a financial provider and then the job is done. Men have always been an active provider to the house and household after their working hours for their wife and children's health, well-being and future as well as maintaining the assets and riches. For example, my grandfather built their own house and made it practical, modern and cosy for his family. He attended all the family dinners and made sure the children ate well. He kept their interest by innovating machines. My other grandpa also attended all the family dinners and he brought the children a sense of religion, social belief and cultural values.

A man that comes home and acts as a guest or a teenager will not survive the marriage or the family for a very long time. It is totally unacceptable physically, mentally and emotional for a woman. It's an illusion to think that this is possible or could have been possible in the grandparent's age or in other religions or cultures. Perhaps it was a little different for the farmers, because their farm was based around their and the women were active on the work terrain. Meals were in the common space and at set timings, this is what makes a family cooperate. The farmer's couple took care of the overall home and business as a joint venture. The children were also part of that overall picture. The woman, in any of these decades and in any family, might or might not have had a job of her own providing or contributing financially. If she doesn't have the extra job, she is certainly spending her hours during the day taking care of her children, the household and the overall continuation of the family. She might be doing this for a few years, a decade or a life time. Day care facilities of the fifties have provided the opportunity for women to hand over their children to other responsible adults and take on industrialized jobs. Basically, the setup is not much different nowadays, but there are usually less children in the household. It's a personal decision and it depends on the financial luxury if a woman or man can remain with the children full-time or part-time. As a matter of fact, the majority of parents would like to spend more time on the responsibility and activities of their children, or simply have time alone to recharge. They can simply not afford it because they need a double income.

Depression and addictions

Imagine a woman is alcoholic and cuts short by a million what she does for her family. Is a female alcoholic acceptable for a family life? A husband might be very patient with such a partner, like a wife would be, but on long term he will never be able to accept an alcoholic, distant wife on the long run. Much like it is unacceptable of a father to be alcoholic and absent. So as mothers, so are fathers, contributing on a daily or weekly basis to their children's physical, mental. emotional, financial and educational wellbeing.

Warning: Unhelpful family and friends are frightened by your fragile situation and can contribute severely to the depression and a couple in distress. The best remedy is that if you are on speaking terms as a couple, to not take any offensive when discussing arrangements with family members and friends that are best for the both of you.

A man that comes home and acts as a guest or a teenager will not survive the marriage or the family for a very long time. You need to show up and step up.

- Andromeda L.C.

Depression creates Anger

This chapter is about reinventing manhood and anger management, bonding issues, neglecting parenthood or fatherhood.

Anger is a creative energy. It's a survival energy to get into action and change a situation. But if we ignore it and ignore our feelings around the anger, it becomes toxic. Toxic for oneself and toxic for others.

Daddy's or partners are extremely worried for the health and pain of their (pregnant) partner, but they are too scared to express this in a caring way, so they suppress. Caring would mean undermining their male ego. I'm saying ego, because it is not the true meaning of 'being a man'. A man is caring, protective, a hunter, ready for action and ready for caressing, ready for giving and ready to take on a danger or responsibility on his 'broad' shoulders.

Daddy's, especially the "Sad Dads", are terrified by the small creature that is a newborn. And for many fathers for the first year the daddy in him doesn't really connect to this creature. Until some "real" communication is sensed or verbal expression and walking which indicate this creature is actually Human Being.

Motherhood, and in that sense fatherhood, is threatening to the Male ego. Even within a woman, her male ego is threatened by Motherhood and will want to survive in some way or another usually by making career and "working hard" to compensate the loss of her becoming a mother.

A Dad Kenny Bodanis wrote a book called Men Get Pregnant Too and there is the Dad 2.0 Summit where Dad Bloggers and Dads gather. That's what being a modern dad is all about. Men are standing up and saying, "I'm a Dad, I'm a parent, I'm equal, I love my kids, I want to care for them and the rest of it, I am human, I can do this. See my fatherhood, it's OK to do the things women do."

The pitfall of Parenthood is Isolation and Depression, the holy grail is Spiritual Enlightenment.

- Andromeda L.C.

Depression creates Isolation

Science and experience are proving that connection, community and creation are the counterparts of loneliness, separation and addiction. Are you feeling lonely, depressed, unproductive, addicted? Create community. A Facebook group, a page, a blog, a twitter hashtag, an instagram account, a gathering, a weekly play group, an online seminar, a neighborhood charity, go to "church" (whatever group that is), join a sport. You have to focus on your purpose, because technology and social media like Facebook will keep you in isolation. It's about connecting, sharing, joining, relating, supporting, common creation, individual effort. An offline community might be an obstacle for you, so the online community is a first step for the ones too isolated in body or mind.

Turn to the people beside you today and build a network of people in a similar situation or people that are like family to you or just with a good or great understanding, even if this is a social worker, therapist or coach. Network.

There are no mom jobs (chores, tasks, responsibilities, roles...), there are no dad jobs, there is just Parenting.

"Men's hormones change during pregnancy and after their babies are born," says Dr. Courtenay. "Pairing those hormone fluctuations with the neuro-chemical changes that occur in the brain as a result of sleep deprivation can combine to create the perfect storm for depression that we see peak in the 3- to 6-month period." says Dr. Courtenay, founder of the website SadDaddy.com.

While a lack of sleep is probably the biggest culprit when it comes depression among new dads, other possible causes include a history of the disease, a dad's rocky relationship with his partner, financial problems or stress, and a sick, colicky, or premature baby. Men who've experienced the loss of loved ones—either in the adult years prior to becoming a parent or while growing up—are also at increased risk for depression.

Internalizing our depression and keeping it to ourselves, is the worst we can do and will effect the partner, the baby and the family as a whole severely. We need to break through the aggressive silence. Silence is also Violence. Your partner might understand your depression, because your partner is in the same situation with a newborn and having children. If your partner is being stubborn about a depressing situation, we need to shake our partner out of it. If this has no effect, we can kindly remind them or guide our partner towards professional help and the support of a family member.

Internalizing depression and internal stress carries a bigger risk to the partner, the couple and the baby. The stress is more likely to come out as violence and aggression.

I think there are two solutions to avoiding and minimizing the post natal depression in both men and women.

1. We need to follow a course in what to expect and learn more about what it means to have children and parenthood. Even if there is no such course available, make this a priority. You can set up your own group, ask a so-

cial worker, your "church" community or even a befriended couple with kids to be openhearted.

2. Expect the you will both suffer from depression, so schedule that you will both see a social worker, psychologist or therapist, doula or someone specialized from the hospital as the arrival approaches and most definitely after the arrival of baby.

These actions will prepare you mentally and emotionally for what is to come and they will prepare a stronger foundation in yourself and with your partner in order to deal with this life transformation. There will be more space or openness to talk about the struggles and depression. There will also simply be more knowledge about the mother's changing body and the care of a baby, which will way heavy on both the man and the woman.

Getting help, taking control of oneself.

If you think your partner or a loved one is suffering from this form of depression, encourage them to get help for everyone's sake.

Dr. Courtenay. "Research consistently shows that a father's postpartum depression has a negative and long-term impact on the psychological, social, and behavioral development of his children—especially boys. We see this in children as young as two, all the way through adolescence, and into young adulthood. This remains true, regardless of whether the mother is depressed. If both parents are depressed, the child's development is even more severely disrupted."

> Your child is not in control of YOUR emotions. It's very scary for a child to think that they would be. You own your own feelings and emotions.
>
> - Conscious Parenting

Depression is a medical condition and can easily be healed, but left untreated it is likely to stay and provoke consequences. Also, the child will not miraculously disappear or change. Having children has its daily struggles for the years to come.

In Becoming A Father, author Dr. William Sears shares his own story of maturing into fatherhood and the important work of raising children.

> You think they reflect on their behaviour (when you shout on them), but it makes them change themselves. They will change themselves to not make others angry.
>
> - Conscious Parenting

Daddy's role

Nursing can be a special bonding time that typically only mother and baby share. Dad can feel left out or disinterested. Sometimes, in order for Dad to have intimacy with Baby too, families make a choice to have Dad sometimes bottle-feed, rather than Mom always breastfeeding.

Nursing can be a bonding time for the whole family. Here is a lovely and bonding way for Dad to be involved in nursing. Sit or lie in a comfy place big enough for all three of you. Have Dad behind or beside Mama so she can lean against him. Dad and Baby may be able to comfortably see each other; but if Baby doesn't look up that far, it is okay-not looking at you doesn't mean your support does not impact Baby.

Maryska Bigos, director of Body-Mind Centering® Infant Developmental Movement Educator trainings, says: "I always encourage Dads to have their own skin-to-skin time with their child by being responsible for bathing with their infant whenever a bath is necessary. It is important after the pregnancy and birth that Dads not let a feeling of being left out discourage them. Be patient and persistent at finding comfortable nursing in side-lying as well as laid-back positions that include Dad (and siblings) in this important family time. At the most basic level, supporting and loving your child's mother is the most effective way to love your child."

As siblings love to interrupt the breastfeeding time, they might as well try having this quiet time with mother and baby lying on the bed. If you get lucky, both children will sleep. You can also have your partner spend quality time with the older sibling, if your partner is around on the weekends or works from home.

How to avoid depression in the first year, Early Childhood and beyond, also for Dads:

- Social Support System
- Hire help at home (nurses, cleaning maids..)
- Seek a Collaborative Relationship with your Partner
- Good Self-Care at all times
- Have weekly quality one-on-one time between daddy and baby by joining a class with other parents.
- Find a babysitter ahead of time, schedule date nights
- Sleep schedule, rest and nap time, even if it is only your eyes, ears or head
- Schedule regular appointments with social workers
- Exercise! Find a new sport or sporty activity to start alone or with a class
- Take Vitamin supplements, especially Magnesium and Vitamin B
- Regulate sleep: both get a smart- or sports-watch with a sleep app
- Order in meals, recipe boxes and store frozen meals (either self prepared, by family or from a good brand).

- Have family and friends on a schedule for eating at their house or sharing their dinner.
- Listen to music and watch Netflix

Talk Therapy, separately and each with his/her own professional if you are going through this "alone" rather than "together", at a psychologist, preferably at a specialized psychologist or therapist for postpartum or new parents. After a few sessions your partner can join your session. If you have the feeling of "being in this together" you can go to a social worker, councillor for new parents, a group or a course. But usually with Postpartum the psychological aspects and relationship problems are bigger and need therapy and treatment.

In the worst case, medications can be a temporary relief to get back on track but they might also provoke other things like more panic attacks if it's not the right one or too heavily dosed for you. So be careful and follow up on it daily for any adjustments. Most hospitals have a psychiatric department where you can stay a few nights or longer period of time in order to heal from sleep deprivation, restlessness and daily pressures. Also consider living in with a family member to get the support and the rest you desperately need. You can work on your relationship. marriage and family life once you both feel better and more stable again.

The difficult part about postpartum or any depression is that the person experiencing it is usually intertwined in him- or herself and therefore not reachable by the partner neither by other individuals. But the partner will suffer from this the most as he / she will be dealing with stress, anger and anxiety outbursts along with guilt tripping and blame. The retrieval, social isolation and perhaps a social mask at your best times, make it difficult for 'outsiders' and especially friends to detect that something is wrong and you need them to really help you by reaching out, giving practical support and pushing you to go seek professional help.

If you can, each on his own, avoid a break up in finding the connection and building the relationship with your baby by the daily caring of your baby, it will avoid another problem on top of the postpartum depression.

It may be helpful to join a support group where you'll meet parents in the same situation. When you're feeling low, it can be hard to get out and about, so an online contact can work for the group. The trick is to stay in touch over the 6 months that you are at risk.

5 Life Hacks

Spare your sanity, don't skip on goodies and baby gadgets

In his chapter I will give you a list of gadgets that guys like to search for and buy, so let him (if you are a female reader)! This is his way to take care, bond with his baby and take care of you.

Gadgets:

- Baby stroller
- Baby seat
- Bottle warmer (my husband's ultimate favorite!), but not a breast pump or food processor!

- Baby husher
- Baby Cam
- Photo Camers
- Smart watch
- iPad or other tablet
- Apps
- Shoes
- Online shopping for deals
- Bargaining Second Hand Items
- His first helicopter, drone or car and other toys from the boy's department

Now, let's look at other life hack tips, which you can make a head start with before baby arrives.

Declutter your house.

Make choices of how you want your house to be supportive of you and your family. These will be the new way of designing your home in order to support your newly grown family unit and your individualism within that unit. An inspiring environment with some artwork, design and such will uplift your spirits and make the nurturing job a whole lot more pleasant on your five senses. It will make it more fun actually. It is not always feasible or necessary, but if you are sensitive to it, it's definitely worth spending your money on design and the cute stuff from the very start. I used to be into second hand clothing and toys, but when the years passed I was more distracted by it and seemed out for a more sleek setup of everything concerning our household.

Decluttering and adding a personal touch is one of the biggest favors you will do for yourself, although it will take a lot of time, energy and even money if you didn't already have the natural ability to be organized and sleek. You might not have the tendency to have an organized house or lack the right furniture. In any case you can look out for tips or help from a friend or even a professional to help the progress of this personal skill. I can see that having at least art work on your walls can save your sanity. The soothing effect and distraction from other mess can really pull you through the day, whereas it had never mattered that much before you had children. Art in a house has a purposeful function: it detracts and inspires the eye to a level where it should be and not on your furniture and mess sitting on the floors.

A child comes with a lot of stuff, clothing, furniture, toys and kitchen arrangements. You will need a budget for children's items because they are priced expensive in the market and even though there are alternatives, they will usually not live up to the design and practical use. However, a child and having a family will take over the household as you knew it and you will become more demanding of everything in your household although their is a strain and lack of time due to the new workload. Making good investments and decluttering from the start will help you to build up a fort where you can all be happy and functional. When you invest in toys for the first year, it is best to invest in wooden toys, bigger attractions (like stations and musical toys) and seats that accommodate the right month in the first two years. Later on, it is best to invest in durable building blocks of all sorts and craft materials.

Avoid the pharmacy when you can

The bills at the pharmacy will stack up, even for small amounts or non-medicated products like cremes, pacifiers and solutions that you think you might need. Or solutions for small ailments, which could have been prevented with more care from the start. Many pharmacies have done their research for natural alternative products in the market, you need to always ask for the healthier alternative and they are happy to show it to you. Not all pharmacies are the same, so keep testing for that one that has more stock of healthier and more herbal medications. In order not to overmedicate your baby, each time you will want to re-ask the same question: what is the healthier alternative? The natural alternative is less harmful to your baby and will heal the baby as fast. These alternatives can be cremes made from nature, homeopathic drops, an oil or an alternative care taking approach to the actual problem. The problem might be a hygienic problem, not a medical one, so the solution is to take care of the hygiene and not of the symptoms. The natural options are usually a quicker way to heal, because it doesn't cover up the symptoms nor does it create side effects. There are many natural ways and solutions to be found in your kitchen in order to heal and sooth. You will find this wisdom on the go, in books or online and with your grandparents solutions.

Both medical and alternative request a lot of information, logic approach and research, so you might as well go for the "alternative", healthy route, instead of the overdressed and surgical route which the majority of parents tend to take. Surgery is not a solution. It is an intervention. And if your baby was not born with this medical situation, it is most likely something that can be healed through alternative medicine (which is not actually alternative, it is natural), through diet, nutritional supplements, different care taking approaches, love, care and such. Start getting in touch with yourself and your own health and wealth, because it will be a life long learning journey and investment in your family's wellbeing. Unfortunately many of us or many Western cultures have lost the wisdom of our grandparents, because they didn't teach us or we weren't documenting it. You might find a book or two about the old, wise, solutions from nature and for your home. This natural route is a preventive route. Regularly feeding and bathing your child in olive and nut oils and a general hygiene, love and care as well as the outdoors will keep your child fit.

Other tips for a practical family home

Meals:

- Take on a cleaning lady twice per week for a few hours so you can spare yourself the dirty household work and spend more time on groceries, cooking and relaxation. It is no luxury once you have decided to go for it.

- Buy a Presto, Crock pot, Grill Machine, Steaming Machine or something that turns food into a meal without actually being present to cook (not a mircowave) if you are not into over dishes

- Make oven dishes or freeze meals, cook double or triple quantities to freeze or keep the remaining meal for the evening or the next day.

- Focus all your groceries on vegetables, fruits, grains, nuts and oils. These are your main food intake. Even if you come home with "only" that, it will feed your family for the next weeks.

- Go for different separate grocery shoppings depending on the purpose of what you need. Shop for vegetables, baby, father, mother, siblings, household separately!

- Cut up fresh vegetables and freeze them, either in separate bags or as a premix if you have liked that particular mix (like a mix of onions, peppers and leak). This is more effective than trying to find your proper brand of vegetables in the frozen section and getting them nicely cooked

- Make different stocks each time you cook up vegetables, fish or meat. Label and freeze them. They add on nutrition, a meaty (or fishy or savory) flavor even if there is no meat as well as variety to upcoming meals, such as rice, couscous, quinoa, beans or as a soup They are far, far more healthier and less salty than a dry bouillon block.

- Freeze fresh sauces for pasta and spaghetti, especially tomato sauce, which kids love and is healthier when it comes from a glass jar rather than a paste.

- Do meal planning, especially if it involves fish or meat, and stick with some meatless staples like beans, brown rice and one or two add on sauces for those "unplanned meals" or lunches. These are ideal kid's meals and really don't need to contain animal proteins every day. The sauce can be enriched with small pieces of meat, chicken or fish every few days if you are semi-vegetarian and IF they don't mind eating it at that meal. Most toddlers are very picky and should be asked if they mind the extra "pieces" in their dish. In this case it is best to keep the meat or chicken in separate frozen portions for add ons. This will also promote making vegetarian dishes which is cheaper for you and environmental- and animal friendly. Kids don't eat big chunks of meat.

- Focus on Vitamin C and if your child has constipation focus on Vitamin C and fibre. Vitamin C is a child's most important building block. They will usually get enough salt from their natural (or industrialized) foods and do not like the taste of added salts.

- If you want to make a sauce or a dish more savory for your tot or your child, you can add on Brewer's Yeast powder. Or if you are cooking up a beans, it can be a fresh vegetable stock from your freezer. Don't add on salt to your cooking. Vitamin C, which children don't mind eating is current in oranges, pressed oranges, kiwi and a few licks of lemon. For long term Vitamin C and fibre they need a few portions of vegetables per week. Every time you need to feed your baby, tot or child focus on either the fruit they can eat or the vegetables they can eat. This requires enough creativity and preparation as is. Other meals will be more staple as mentioned: beans, brown rice and an add on. This doesn't need to be a mix for toddlers, because they usually want their ingredients separate and organized on their plate.

- Focus on "the vegetable of the day" or "cuisine of the day" and make variations to that vegetable or cuisine.

- Decide on five family dinners and five family lunches and always stick with these meals. This way you will have good expectations, tasty dishes and not to mention; less visits to the grocery store.

- Order your groceries online, make it your basic list, so you can repeat this grocery list each week until the season changes.

- Stock up on really good boxes for in your fridge and storage cabinets. Store all possible grains and superfoods each in a separate box, so you can easily choose it as an add on to your fruits or veggies. Store in your fridge snack size and peeled fruits, boiled eggs, chicken legs, olives and cut up veggies. Store in your freezer cut up potatoes for fresh french fries, soups and sauces. Store in your fridge a box of cooked up spaghetti, cooked up rice and just add on as you please with a sauce or some other toppings. The point is: the system will help you to prep or cook food. Having a recipe book will not.

Toys:

- Buy 50% of your toys in wood, especially blocks, blocks and blocks. These are the prettiest in your household, non-toxic and kids love playing with blocks. There are some truly amazing building blocks on the market! Unless cars, dolls, and Lego, these will enrich your home environment and the intelligence of your child.

- Invest in baskets, woven basket, or something that pleases your eye to burry up the toys effectively and quickly. These baskets will enrich the play area and your living space.

- Set up stations of toys according to the activity. Much like a nursery. You can have a station for the water colors, another for the building blocks and another for a dress up party. Depending on the space in your house, you can have different corners depending on the activity. Books and teddybears are in the bedroom, the play corner is in the living area, the color station in the kitchen and the dress-up party in your bedroom. It will help you to play different interesting activities throughout the day or the week and keep your child more interested in a variation of activities instead of resorting to the t.v. Each station can be enriched with its own challenge depending on their age and growth. You will come up with your own creativity and symbolic meanings in your life, which makes it your play as much as their play.

Clothing:

- Buy wrinkle free clothing, not too tight on your body so it will adapt to your size and last for the next half decade

- Buy leggings and such stretchy pants for your babies and children, even if they are boys. It grows with them for the next 3 years and they can play in them safely instead of tight buttoned up jeans which don't stretch and press their bellies. There is one brand I'm currently aware of that does stretchy jeans and there are usually legging jeans available for girls, which again can work for boys. It also makes more sense for potty training and they can fall asleep with it and go out the next day. It will save both parent and child frustrations while getting dressed and undressed in the years to come. Simply, don't buy button up jeans or pants.

- Don't buy new clothing for yourself in the first year postpartum, your body and looks will change significantly. Make your major investment after at least the first birthday and if you are having a second child, it was probably not worth the investment. Your style will change again as you gracefully mature into a mother.

- Do small washes rather than big ones. Look for the express mode (20 minutes) on your machine and the extra centrifuge round to dry clothing out before hanging them to dry.

- Bring shirts to iron or dry-clean to a shop. All important adult (and kids) clothing can be cared for outside of the home so you need to was only the baby and indoor clothing.

- Take on your most precious baby items through carry-on luggage, in case you will lose your baggage.

- Lend clothing for your baby and buy second hand clothing and second hand products and shoes at summer fairs in the summer time. Hit those seasons with the garage sales and don't skip on items. This is if you are into second hand, preloved items at all for baby and otherwise it can work for you when the child is older and you need to watch a budget. Personally I've always like the authentic style of the items I could find for a fraction of the price of shop items.

- Some countries offer a subscription for trendy, new clothing which grows with your child and the seasons for a fixed price per month.

- Clothing at a market fair or in a voluntary store will be even cheaper than a private garage sale or a privately owned second hand shop. Shoes are harder to find, so shop them ahead if you don't mind buying second hand or buy them in sale for a summer or winter ahead.

- Shop for seasons and years ahead, it will come quicker than you think. Make matching outfits. Stick to 3 colours for yourself and your children.

- Let your child, starting somewhere at age 2-2,5 years pick his own clothing. At this age they start having a preference for some kind of cartoon on their clothing and they have their own preference of style, both boys and girls. You can still dress them up without cartoons on a festive day or party, but on regular days, why not let him wear the shirt he picks or the dress she picks. So avoid overbuying or buying what they don't like by letting them simply shop and choose themselves at a young age!

- Keep the clothing and toys that don't give you a good feeling in a box or bag and look onto them in a few months. If you are still not finding a good purpose to keep them among your daily belongings, get rid of them by giving them to a good cause or shelter.

- Storage also costs money, even if it's in your own home. It costs you time, energy and a bigger house. So think about the space you want to stay with in your house, because a bigger house will demand and gather more stuff. If you want to live cosy or minimalist, you need to stick with a smaller house and perhaps more outdoor living area. More furniture and stuff also means more storage system and extra costs when moving them to a new house.

Hygiene:

- Use a dry shampoo to replace the shower for your hair. You might have to test a few, but then you will find one that will work for you and if it is enough organic you can use it on your toddler for those times they refuse to wash their long hair or you just don't have time for the hassle.

- Use an authentic sea sponge for cleaning those baby and toddler bums instead of wet wipes or other. It is extremely effective and environmental friendly. You can have a second sponge for cleaning the body. This sponge is extremely hygienic, soft, effective and suitable for washing of poo. For the face I like to use small square face towels which are soft and tend to dry more quickly than the usual wash cloth.

Groceries:

- Let your basic groceries be delivered home or set aside at the pickup of the supermarket.

- Let a weekly or two-weekly recipe package be delivered to your house. These packages contain the exact measurement of ingredients for a homemade recipe.

- Order the products you love online and have them delivered. Know your apps and become a smart online buyer.

- Cut open end of tubes to get to another reservoir of toothpaste to save yourself a shopping trip and buying expensive toiletries. Get potty trained quickly and have diaper free days at home to cut down on the expense and environmental waste. Use cloth diapers if you can.

Items:

- Keep the boxes, instructions and batteries of all your baby products so you can sell them decently to new mothers.

- Keep the receipts and the instructions of purchases in a ziplock bag in one place for later reference and guarantees. You will need them to refresh on how to use the product in different phases and for your own guarantee when things break down. A new client for your product will want to have the guidelines for a quick look into buying, especially if the instructions are not available online.

- Buy festive ornaments, gifts and birthday decorations out of season so you can buy them on a discounted price and ahead of time, not in a last minute rush because you are now celebrating family events.

- Donate toys to other children of friends to refresh their set of toys for the next week(s) and donate other clothing and items to charity. Lots of families need help and a boost. It will also teach yourself and your children to help out others and society. It takes an effort and once you know your way, it does not take an effort, it is so rewarding. We need to find our way to the charity in order to hand over the goods. No matter what our income, we can all share in our wealth much more than we are willing to admit.

- You can rent an official electric pump for expressing milk or make the investment in a double electric pump that expresses from both breasts; these pumps are far more effective than any electric hand pumps from the store. Making the extra investment for a double one, can mean winning time and energy if your breasts express milk at the same time and if there is a lot of milk to express.

6 Unleashing the Tiger Mom

From maiden to momzilla

The mother of mothers is celebrated and is guiding us, in the form of Goddess Yemoja and Mary Magdalena amongst many others.

Your baby has arrived. You are now a mother. Although you won't feel like one right away, that is pretty sure. Being a mother comes with experience and some women will feel it sooner, others later. Some may take years and others never will. There is one thing for sure: you are no longer the innocent daughter of the universe or daughter in law to anyone anymore. You entered the game of Motherhood and Moms Rivalry. You have come to a point of criticism and might be left lonely and disheartened. Why are they mean? Why haven't they warned me before? Why am I going through this passage? What have they done to me? Is this the lonely planet I now belong to? Mombie Planet. Until you figure out that, not everyone has exactly the same pressure or experience, but there are other mombies out there and you share more than one or few things in common. You are not alone on this journey. There is in that sense a sisterhood in the motherhood. On the streets and the shops, you basically just need to spot another mom with her child and you will become best friends for life! Motherhood; a circle of women who have passed through a passage comprising birthing process, but not acknowledged in the Western society. We become mother, but we are uninformed and unaware. We are "having children" according to Western society and this is all we know and that may or may not be "life changing". So we create, connect, seek ourselves and ultimately each other through social media, coffee mornings, play groups, play dates and other self sought tribes.

Your body is becoming a mommy (or mombie), your soul is becoming a mommy (or mombie), your mind is becoming a mommy (or mombie), you are becoming a mommy (or mombie) holistically. It takes time though, perhaps years and perhaps someone will never embrace the evolution of becoming a mother. With the years and our spiritual evolution we evolve from one being to another on a scale of wisdom and life experience. We birth ourselves into mothers after being maiden and with age we can become an Enchantress, usually around the age of 40-50 years and a

Crone around the age of 60 years. Don't expect to go back and don't wish to go back. You never will. Life is pushing you forward. As much as you never will go back to being a baby girl, a fiancee, a maiden, or a young mother, you will never go back in evolution. And if you cannot embrace it, you are missing a part of your power and magic. And you are stealing from your child, children at whole and society by not giving that what evolution has to offer.

These transformations are a permanent one that can bring you much beauty and wisdom. You can align and update yourself to a trendy, sexy, savvy and confident mom for sure, but the beauty and wisdom counts. It will take normally at least a year to year and a half postpartum to get in your own body and mind, rather than being the vehicle of your baby. It might take 2, 3, 4, 6, 10 years to get to a place you feel comfortable and empowered in to replenish yourself and your new body and role whether that is at the stage of mother, enchantress or the crone.

The sooner the better though, because these stages evolve around self-love and self-care and it is always a good time for self-love and self-care. We are asked to feed ourselves and to have a good night rest. Give yourself that time or consciousness needed! Although it will not come easily and sufficiently in the first half year, we somehow manage or make a breakthrough on the good and bad habits to become a healthier vehicle and mothership for our children and ourselves.

The mothership and being the taxi-driver

You might also invite your Inner Child to board the mothership, as your inner child is already there, but can be tendered to much more willingly. This is the process of unraveling and unlearning, un-teaching yourself, the so called 'wooliness' of society which wasn't much wool at all. Especially if you consider the rotten feelings you encounter and the individualistic lifestyle you are now destined to live within a strange and cruel world.

We've lost our ways of tribal living, our children as well. Them too are living individualistic lives. They don't get the comfort of growing up surrounded with other children and adults, other than parents and siblings, if they live isolated from family connections. Especially in the early years, when mother spends most of her time indoors, she can feel the lack of a tribe and the tribal living which other (ancient) civilizations and ancient times offer. We occupy our children with activities and taxi rides to their friends, as they grow up, in order to give them more of a social life and occupation.

Motherhood is a career. You cannot get there with just few months or few years of experience. This is also what you should tell your partner or family member when they are going down the path of criticism. Other moms just might have 10, 20, 30, 40 years more experience than you. That means they have more inherent, natural abilities and skills for routine, program, prepping food, feeding, playing, bed time, kid's psychology, family planning, finance and such. Also, they might on their turn be great at one aspect and failing miserably on other points, wishing their children were better fed, or rested, or supported, or educated, or socialized.

Overall, the long-term moms had a better chance to get things right in their household and to make healthy cooking a tradition. The lunch boxes are a PhD on its own. The family units of the dinosaur moms are like a strong fort, they've built onto it each single year. Also, when your children are still in diapers or just very young, you cannot measure yourself to a family that has children of a bigger age group. You will get to that stage and flexibility when your babies have grown up to that age group and when they are less physically and emotionally dependant on you for living life.

Don't rush yourself and especially don't drive yourself crazy. You are really doing a great job getting by and learning on the way how to better things. It's really a phase. A damned one. A phase that both partners need to accept and expect. Having babies for the first time or having a baby after your other kids are grown up is not easy and it's hectic in time and energy management. You might have the experience as a mom, but your postpartum pregnancy and baby will not be different from the first one. Like my friends in The Netherlands have told us: those young years are the tropical years.

Give yourself that time and ask this time from your partner and relatives. As I'm finishing this book (or think I am) and heading for the 2nd birthday (now 4th birthday) of my son, I can tell you I'm nowhere near feeling like a trendy, sexy, savvy and confident mom. I went through an emotional crisis wondering if I should still be living at home, in my marriage or if I was going to make it on my own. I went through more than a year of insomnia and hard 24/7 work followed by a period of trying to recuperate, to be hit by a mental imbalance of brain chemistry. The sleep deprivation, pressure, hard work and stress was getting the better of me after the first one and a half year of baby. I felt I was literally going crazy and so I decided to be hospitalized for a few nights. My husband couldn't help me at this point, as any husband or wife can lose their partner to an illness, addiction or depression. Such was I. It was for a few nights with a few medication to slow down my hyperactivity, but I might as well have stayed for a long period of time or be truly hit by a chemical imbalance for the long term. I can imagine this has happened to women and men. I can imagine this is truly how healthy, productive people actually turn crazy. Besides, depression runs in one part of my parent's family. Despite all this, I know I'm on the track of being a mom that found her new path in life and is loved by her child(ren). The rest will sort itself out by balancing the healthy foods, with Netflix and some order-in pizzas and burgers. Food for thought! Don't underestimate your diet and nutrition as a parent, it takes on a life of its own. A nutritional focus helps me effortlessly through the days and an intuitive clean eating keeps me well fed, balanced with some fatty foods, meat and homey dishes once in a while. We need to keep up with such a high performance sport!

Being the rock

Back to the baby. Those first weeks and months at home can give some moments of insecurity, even with the second or third baby, because it brings along new tasks, stress and dynamics to the current family member (even your pets). I would tell my husband on the first baby to "be like a tree" or to "be like a rock", a safe haven for the baby to cling onto emotionally. When you imagine and feel this emotion, the baby can actually hold on to you morally. If you are trembling like a leaf, it also effects your long term endurance. I remember how Raphael one time in his life slept his head on a shoulder, and it wasn't even mine. It was the shoulder of a police officer at my sister's FBI job. The woman had a sturdy, friendly posture and adored holding a child in her arms. This reflected on the baby and responded to that by clinging on to her chest to relax. Somehow, he is and was not the feely, touchy baby and could literally hold himself independent. The kind of security and confidence you want to seek as a parent, is the kind you will want and need for the months and years to come. You and your children will feel uplifted when you can be trees and boulders. It will be a wonderful gift to your baby and children as they grow up. I was always self confident, at least, I thought in my mind I was, but to feel like the actual rooted and strong tree didn't come until I had three years and a whole lot of self-appreciation accomplished in my mom career. And I'm still only mom of a three and one year old.

No holidays, only over hours

Becoming a parent is like taking on a full-time job with many over hours and no holidays. There are many insecurities, questions and frustrations to deal with. It remains. Although it comes in moments of crisis and it dissolves when practicing conscious parenting, I hardly think it will ever really pass because the family life is constantly evolving. I'm not sure if parents ever feel settled for long because it demands a whole lot of self confidence and self control to figure out yourself, your children, your marriage, your household, your activities and business and so on. It is possible though. In the course of four years I've settled with many or all aspects with parenting, a little less with working my own hours away from my babies and with other people. In order to make your weakness your strength, you have to go through the shit of it (literally). I bet you have literally or metaphorically shitted your pants on some occasions or subjects of parenthood. How to organize life between work, time off and the child(ren) is a big part of that equation. One wonders how so many parents pull it off, especially in the individualistic societies and economies we live in. School schedules and school holidays every 6 weeks v.s. a work schedule are one mind boggling exercise! I haven't figured it out yet and I'll be a stay at home mother and freelancer as long as I haven't figured it out. Part of our family moving to the Middle-East is the easy, affordable and trustworthy access to a full-time nanny and/or other helpers for cleaning and babysitting. And yet, you might not have that access, it is important to keep in mind that it is a phase and that each new phase will give new opportunities for you to have more time and energy for you, work and time off. Every family unit is a different unique organism and you simply cannot copy and paste it. You cannot even copy your own parents, as life will present you with similar karmic challenges but with different perspectives, qualities and dynamics. Go figure.

It is so freakin' messy! Try Stain' Alive!

It gets messy. Not only in the house, but in your life in general. Your new job and role as parent takes a lot of time getting used to and maybe never does, like any other dynamic and high performance job? Kids are simply not objects; they are in constant motion and extremely needy by their nature and nurture. You're always on top of it and many times dwelling under the mess and the stress that goes with it. If you don't want to do the dirty work and get your hands in it full time, think twice about "having a child". You will be sacrificing yourself, your life and your house to your child, even if you made yourself believe a different version of parenthood as I describe in this book. I'm trying to give you the truth of it, the break-down, without the sarcasm of it (which makes for great jokes, you will find them in plenty!). Children need 24/24 hours surveillance by adults. And they all say: big children, big problems. So, let's see. I still believe I will be fine with that because I have already "psycho-managed" the relationship from the start, but yes, when they annoy you for not being the 'sweet little angel that does what you want or expect', how are you going to balance out all your frustrations, time, stress, and worries about your child and your lack of everything to manage it? This is why the qualities of consciousness and conscious parenting gives so much peace.

Babysitting; a trouble to find and finance

Be the Buddha or else seek for it. So the sleepless nights are not just reserved for the baby years. What does that mean for your current day and night schedule? Unlike a cat or a dog or any other pet, your children will not be left 5 minutes on their own in their baby years and not 50 minute alone in the house until maybe 10 years of age. If you are not spending your own time on your child(ren), then that means someone else is babysitting them. Be it your parents, parents-in-law, daycare or a nanny or a combination of them. Most parents rely on programs and services organized for their children starting at the crib, the kindergarten, the school, the after-school activities, the summer camps just to fill up all those minutes, hours, days, weeks of "having children". Sure, they need a social life, education and play time. But still: we have babies and than we work to find all the babysitting solutions to fill up the days of the week. Not me, but I mean, "you" in general right? Some will seek more part-time solutions and others will seek full-time solutions, whatever it is, you will need it in order for you and your children to survive and evolve. Again, the summer holidays and other holidays are devastating to parents. Who is going to stay with them all those days? Parents, actually, can hardly live a couple of weeks without those programs and services to assist them. Both on a financial and emotional level. Ask parents about the "summer holidays", they have a totally different meaning for parents. It means literally the 2 months when school is closed, not your beach vacation. As a matter of fact, many beach vacations have been more stressful to parents than staying around their neighborhood. You will get the seriousness of this mind boggle once you get out of the maternity years or the first half year of care. Being a 24/7 parent is nearly impossible. I'm telling you so by experience of being a Stay At Home Mother. And regarding the fact you need your time off, you just don't get it. It's the number one complaint of most moms and the dads seem not to jump in as a babysitter once in a while for the mom to relax her mind and body or see her friends (alone) for just a bit. Hence, going to the supermarket alone (when dad does give you a break) is the ultimate Bali trip and a spa haven for a new mom. So if you're doing the job alone, you will need a part-time day care sooner or later but the need is the highest around month 7. Some mothers will be better able to be a full-time SAHM doing the job alone than others. My best friend didn't consider a day care at all even if she had one full year of a non-sleeping and awfully crying baby, when I was actually desperate for some solution by month 11 and never had a crying baby (sleepless, yes). I had gone through so much emotional drama in my relationships, maybe it made the difference. But it's normal that a person would ask for some time off. Other mothers wouldn't survive more than a few weeks or few months. It all depends on the person, the situation and how much you are willing to take. However, you desperately need to get honest and find the right balance somehow for you and your baby because you will go insane. In my case I developed a chemical imbalance in my brains, due to 1,5 year of all kinds of stress including... this list is too long. Thank God our physical health was top fit and there were no actual deaths in the family. It was only insanity. At that moment I ran out to the hospital where I had both my babies born and asked for help at the emergency. With several nights of rest and actual medications to slow down the race and imbalance my body and brains were in, I managed to get back on track over the days, weeks and months. Watching 7 seasons of Pretty Little Liars, which my husband was happily to assist in me being glued to the couch, was my savior over the long term of 6 months. A few caring people in my life and a professional bunch of social workers were the reason I was saved on the shorter and mid-long term. When you really need it, you will find the help you desperately need and haven't been asking, getting or receiving from the beginning. I'm your shining example of possibilities. It is all possible. Nothing is IM-possible and a lot of it again depends on the choices you make, the decisions you take and how much you are willing to take. Sacrifice is a big part of the momhood. It is not a fairy tale life as we imagine it by our oblivious minds.

> **Welcome to Motherhood.**
> **Welcome to getting in touch with a new you.**
>
> - Andromeda L.C.

What about Women's PSTD?

Men tell stories where women get panic attacks and show a lot of anger and rejection, while the men who love them, want to hold on to them, be close to them and tell them how they love them. Yet, the woman is rejective, hostile and "out of her mind". Yes, there are women that fell into illness and there are men out there suffering from their ill partner, not knowing what to do about it. PSTD will happen, no matter what. It is not a question of 'some women get PSTD and will it happen to you or your friend?'. The question is: how severely will you get it and for how long?

I choose not to talk extensively about PSTD in women for several reasons:

1. Every new mother (also second or third time mothers) will go through a lot of physical challenges and changes including healing and hormonal adjustments, paired with new experiences, bonding and sleeping problems, burn outs, daily challenges, long term commitments, financial issues, personal achievement issues etc, etc, etc. A normal person

would go through depression for less than that. Luckily Moms have a super power to keep them (somewhat) alive and kicking. Unfortunately due to physical inner and outer challenges, women are pushed or fall into a depression of some sort. This could be an accumulated fatigue resulting into hormonal imbalance and this could be an hormonal or other chemical disturbance right after birth causing the mother to be off the chart and rejecting her child (as well as partners or other children).

2. I didn't experience it as such. I felt perfectly fine, happy and healthy in my brains, in my body and in relationship with my babies. Hindsight I can see that PSTD for me comes out in shadows of myself and is reflected in my relationships and that I live in a brain bubble for a year which feeds the intimacy of maternity for body and soul. So yes, I experienced it, but I didn't feel it as such to give it enough importance or for people to acknowledge that I am a source of problems.

3. Mothers' problems, and therefor big part of society's problems, are too often blamed on mothers being "crazy" under the influence of their hormones and the isolation they live in.

4. PSTD is a medical disease and as it progresses in more severe cases it is an illness, that needs close followup by professionals, loved ones, healing and some medications to assist if taken responsibly. This illness separates the child from it's mother in order to be taken care of and remain in safety when the mom is at risk. Some countries like Belgium have recently opened a new department for their hospitals in order to take in mothers and their babies for

full-time care of their PSTD and relationship and functional problems whilst caring for their infant. I strongly encourage every hospital to extend their services from prenatal to postnatal followup and not only for the women that suffer, but as a proactive treatment, because birth (from pregnancy to breastfeeding) by nature is traumatizing for our bodies and brains.

Feminine is Rising in men as well

It's time to find back female energy. Feminism is often misunderstood by both women and men, or interpreted in a way that strives for strong, somehow independent from men or lesbian women. Feminism in a more true sense is about equality and for everyone to be empowered and balanced in their choices. Divine Feminine is about the female energy in each of us that needs balancing with the male dominated energy and structure we live in. Energy stand for both the male and the female energy that possesses our bodies and souls. Finding back female energy is about balancing the male qualities and the female qualities so we can feel and be more whole. More sane actually. When we 'think we are going crazy' we are actually trying to balance out the male and female energy.

Our society is male dominated, which means both men and women are robbed of their feminine energy and qualities. Men are not allowed to cry, to be weak, to care, to be emotional, to do the fine arts, to be hugged, to be kissed, and so on. Gay men are stoned to death either literally or emotionally. So please, it is not all about the women here. Modern day society is actually somewhat a good place for women! They have a chance to be strong, modern, independent, free and achieve. They have a chance to be like a man. Only to discover that, both man and women, are too manly and we are missing the other part of ourselves. And we are missing the relaxation, receptivity and recreation, which are all feminine qualities of being human. Still, many women have marriage and family as an ideal, which is not an awfully feminine or feminist goal if you ask me. You can create and grow family, but it needs tweaking of the mind and values in order to stay alive and have an updated version of the woman's role in marriage.

Feminism is about empowering that part of us that makes us weak and for the weaker among us not to be hidden from the society or the respect of our eye. The weak are our children but also elderly, disabled, the weirdo and pretty much everyone that differentiates from the idealized Hollywood man or woman. It even include the criminals.

Competing women

Women fail being true to their womanhood. It is a big disappointment in people you could face even if it was already part of your life before. The competition, jealousy and logic reasoning wins from their sensitivity, understanding and sisterhood. Your mom (and mom in law) have been a mom too for maybe 2,3,4,5,6 times in a row. But they also forgot a big part of it and they became someone else, perhaps someone bitter. The mind doesn't keep up with what we were doing the last year, let alone 10 - 40 years ago. The same will happen to you. You will have a hard time remembering and relating to the time and the person you were, when your baby was a new born by the time it is crawling, walking, talking.

Unless you make a heartfelt connection and step in the shoes of a caretaker, it will again be difficult to understand or help another young mother. Can't she just do it and be normal? This is the main reason in many cases you can count only on professional help when you are in maternity and a doula arranged around your delivery. Naturally or hopefully you will count on the father of the baby. Everyone else is a welcome addition, but needs some evaluation and they should come into your new life with a big, forgiving, heart in order to not break down the newly created family. Even if intentions and care taking is excellent, it might still weaken a family unit if they did not get a chance to do it on their own before the initial 3 months have passed.

These are some professional services you can search for in order to support you and your family member. Also ask your governmental institutions for contacts and support that you are entitled to, such as:

- Cleaning ladies
- A chef that comes at home, groceries delivered at home, order-in menus, subscriptions to food packages, catering services, catering shop with prepped food ('traiteur'), high quality frozen meals
- Psychiatrist, Psychologist, Therapist, Social Worker
- Lactose specialist
- Doula

- Life Coach, Parent Coach, Parent Advisor or Expert
- Kinesist
- Genealogist
- Paediatrician, Children Therapist
- Maternity Nurse, Midwife
- Au pair, Nanny, Babysitting, Family member
- Babysitting and extracurricular programs for older siblings
- Driver or reliable taxi driver

Now I will discuss the 2nd big disappointment: you might not be able to count on the help or understanding of a professional. They too are human and they too can disappoint you in times of uncertainty and fragile health.

You need to see several doctors and speak about your problem, if possible with the father's baby around. I've been let down by at least two doctors when I needed them the most and I was only helped partially by other doctors on several occasions when I was at my most desperate.

It took the big crisis 1,5 year into motherhood where my sanity was failing, for me to becoming able to truly receive help and support on different matters. These previous described disappointments had severe consequences on my health and on my husband's stress and anger levels.

In general, we can say, that if you are not suffering from a visibly physical ailment, if your problems are mental and emotional, you are taken less seriously. And sleep deprivation is not taken seriously. Neither maternity nor relationship problems during parenthood. Actually from a certain point of view, it was better I had not seen a psychologist, because it made family matters worse as I now was officially "crazy and suicidal". It all drove me insane and deteriorated my health, but not until a year and a bit later when I really needed a psychiatrist to medicate me to slow down the fight, flight, freeze reactions of my total system. By society, including family, you are considered normal, healthy, ready and capable of doing your job as a mother, under whatever Godly given circumstance. But that is not entirely true. Doing the mom job with a mom body alone is already the job of a pretty crazy person, but doing that under pressured circumstances such as mental, emotional and financial poverty is just outrageous.

As a new mother, your vulnerable position, sensitive body and severe lack of sleep are no imaginary problems. It might not be respected, but they are there. So be prepared once you come back home with your baby facing the real world. In Belgium and Bahrain we have a standard of couple of nights recuperation in the hospital after delivery, in The Netherlands you get sent home the first day. Check the possibilities in your country and perhaps stay longer in the hospital or make sure the midwives come long hours to your home. The extra time at the hospital is taken for several activities:

- Nursing your wounds

- Following up your health

- Following up your baby's health

- Educating you on baby's care and in some cases breast-feeding (unfortunately not all countries promote and some even discourage a natural feeding)

You can also ask your Doula to visit you after the birth, until you feel you have everything under control.

Trust and the lack of it

Don't give your trust for free now that your role and position has changed within your family's structure. Trust is something that people earn and than deserve, it has to be earned first. Someone that keeps breaking your trust, emotionally, in a practical sense, or both will not be a good friend and probably not a good help towards your family. If a relative, friend or professional is given your trust for free, without a questioning or test phase before or after your delivery, there is a big chance of misuse of power once you become a mother and the consequences will become extremely hurtful to you.

It might sound harsh, and it is, for 'survival of the fittest' can be brutal and cruel to the weak. Take on an attitude of a tiger or lioness to survive this period of time. Than you can win in this wild adventure! You gave birth to your most precious gift of life and the two of you have to be protected from predators. In this game, anyone can be a predator, from your most beloved and trusted ones to the most random people on the street or exes in your exes past. The becoming of a mother, especially the first time around, take some shape shifting. It could happen a second time around, that again changes things completely around.

Your best friend, husband, mother, sister and such might not be your best friend in this period of time. If they are lost-in-translation and negative emotions like jealousy or revenge take over, you might consider not seeing them for the time being. You are not in need of the psychological games on top of your new job. You will come out stronger and maybe wiser once you depend more on your own self-love and take the lessons of life. I know I did. The negativity might also have healed some old wounds and released the skeletons in the closet. But honestly, you don't need it. And I don't wish it to anyone, because I've been through emotional hell on Earth and saw what blame games and divorce scenarios from partners and family are like.

Nowadays I have so much sympathy and compassion for the weaker than me, of all ages and races, especially when abuse and misuse have become a physical practice. The human crime in this world is immense and yet each one of us has their own suffering and wounds to heal, no matter the physical repercussion. I wish we could be sane, be whole and be loved from the start as a baby, we wouldn't need so much conflict and suffering in our soul or the physical abuse and even wars would become less of an agenda, I like to believe. This is part of loving your child(ren) consciously; to safeguard a world of peace. I wish the innocent to be protected from the evil souls and darkness out there hunting our babies, mothers, women, men and our humanity. We can change the spiritual love revolution we are fighting in the West one baby and one parent at a time. The baby needs you and vice versa. Also, you need you more than ever before. The self. That's all that counts. Nothing else counts. We need this kind of Love Revolution until we find green solutions for our global living and ward of the evil. Or perhaps we will transcend, each good soul at a time, but in both cases, we cannot simply sit in our shit. You need not accept that you are part of the negativity towards your inner child, your children and the community. We are in state of desperation to evolve to a better life for the self and a higher consciousness to reside and function from.

For me, having a baby and taking care of him for the first time, was 0% challenge compared to the stress levels, psychological games, negativity and threats that I was experiencing from the "outside world". I've heard a lot of verbal diarrhoea, I guess 100 times more than the actual diapers I had to change by myself. I'm still not clear on what is fact and what is fake of what was said and done. Is it the reality of others or is this my inner demons showing up? I do know and realize, once again, that we do teach people how to treat us, but often unconsciously from our own foundation of life (our Diamond Year). The limits and boundaries we set and the amount of self-love reflect what we will see in the "outside world". Especially the amount of self respect and self- confidence is undermined, even if you think you are doing pretty well, you are not, if you are constantly confronted with shadow selves.

It is your relationships and (conscious) choice of relationships that show your inner world. Once you are in a weak physical position it's too late to teach yourself and others to respect, because the physical world will take over your life to promote your inner world for a real change.

I'm mentioning sub-conscious, because I've managed through training to have a big heap of awareness in my mind and this is what kept me sane in those insane times.

Birthing and maternity was one of the most challenging periods of my life. My sub-conscious had a good foundation and awareness through training and the way of Tao, but it still lacked what it needed most: a change of believes and cutting of the toxicity in and around me. And it's exactly this what can comes out, pops up and starts throwing itself up on you. The whatever you have been keeping from the light over the years, will show up in a midlife crisis to give you a final decision of self-reevaluation, self-transformation and self-actualization. My midlife came at 30-35 years old, instead of 40-45 years of age, and this might very well be the trend for adults. All in all, no adult lives an easy life. Wether single, in relationship, married, divorced, children or no children, once we hit 30's we are dealing with the harshness of our karma in the hope to transform it into dharma.

Maybe it is also Karma being a bitch for all the bad choices you made earlier in life. We all have done bad things to ourselves and others. I was hardly aware of what I had been keeping inside or the level of consciousness I was at to begin with, which was despite my awareness really terribly low on the ladder of self-love and self-actualization.

When you are somewhere on the minus 5 or minus 10, it gets pretty "hellish" and this is where people are suicidal. Unfortunately for them, they might remain in the hell of the realms, because we don't move up the ladder of realms until we have evolved our consciousness. Your inner secrets come out and show their ugly heads. You can have them on a platter, like me, or through bigger life events, such as accidents and illness. Of course we are not all hit by these dynamics in the same way, as many people out there, as many stories. This is just one of the stories which many people can and will find their own truth reflecting in it. You are not alone on this journey and usually all the possible stories are well written about, documented and shared with peers.

Unfortunately, my inner secrets are usually connected to a history, a period of time where I didn't influence much in my life. I was not in control, because I was too young. The history of your conception, your mother's world, your birth process and your youth make up the person and product you have become. Better said: the inner secrets of your parents will pop out. As those from the baby's other parent parents. And this can get ugly. It might even lead to reasons, now or later, for a breakup, separation or divorce. If you can win and battle these inner secrets, you are on a good way of lasting and potential happy family life. Not without problems of course, but they will exist on a familiar level ready to be solved. If they take the better of you, you are headed for more burn outs and divorce, which divorce has not seen the end yet. Divorce does not happen overnight, separation does, but spiritual, practical and financial divorce does not. It can take years and years and it might never resolve if the peace and arrangements do not settle in. The question should be: how does divorce happen to a "happily" "married couple" "having a child"?

For me it al started here:

My delivery process was heavily criticized. I'm not going to elaborate much on this matter, as I believe – and I think the world with me – that a delivery in whatever shape, way or form is not a subject of criticism. Unless my birth it seemed.

Unlike many other subjects around motherhood, the birth is usually not an issue to other people. There is no advice, comments or criticism about the baby you brought to the world, let alone the moment you are pushing out the baby. But mine was, continuously, even during labor a subject of criticism. My or my baby's birth was criticized, for weeks and weeks and weeks at end and then it morphed into other unrelated subject matters as a reaction to the first and so forth and so on. Welcome to my new life. Welcome to the mother role amongst the Maffia. I felt that I really needed a lawyer some time soon to defend my mom-rights. But what rights does a mom have in this world? Close to none, right? Moms are 'crazy bitches'. It can take a long while to find the right people, professionals, friends and family that will stick out for a mom. It is a huge ridicule.

This ridicule is part of what got me back to the hospital after only ten days into postpartum and which made me lose my patience with the subject on several occasions. I tried to anger, ignore, explain, explain again, be patient, reject, resist, persist in my strength and calm,… but nothing seemed to scare the skeletons away.

Even if I was untouched, it only got worse and transformed to new situations for the next year or two to come. I tried to feel more, to express myself more, to stand up for myself more and to find the essence of it. It all failed and I thought again I might need a lawyer, but this time for a separation. After learning my lessons, I can say: I might have been untouched by all the negativity coming my way, I still need to feel and verbalize my boundaries in a more essential way in every word, action and fibre without failure. This is something I haven't learnt in Early Childhood. I always cross my boundaries. The criticism I got from my close ones on birth were:

- I was making the people wait on purpose.
- I was pushing other people's buttons as usual.
- I was a witch during the delivery.
- My baby was proving me wrong.
- I refused to take doctor's advice or medication
- I was suicidal during birth
- I was treating people as a slave
- I was selfish

So, I went to several psychologists, coaches, therapists, healers, social workers and even saw a psychiatrist when I thought I was going crazy: falling into a psychosis. I worked on processing the year's events, the relationship with my mother, hidden emotions from the past recurring in the present, my own birth trauma, stepping into my strength and setting boundaries, letting go of control and the outside world, slowing down and caring for my own, hitting the pause button, sinking into my inner peace, following a path of happiness not of pain.

The therapist that I so adore from pre-partum and revisited for a postpartum family constellation marked the following on my male & female energies and roles:

"I noticed during the session that you were looking to the outside world and getting confused by it. You were not in your power and did not work with your intuition (female energy) rather with your logic and reasoning (male energy). I see a big female presence in you. I want to work with you on finding this, yet for now I'm asking you to sit still and give yourself time to integrate into being a mother, a big part of being woman. In the constellation you are looked at as a woman with big powers en someone that will help to bring the system in balance. Please know that our society is very male dominant which applauds focus, self-preservation and ambition when actually the feminine side deserve more space and existence. For the time being, take healing and cleansing showers of colored light and send back anger issues of red and gold back to the system".

Until the day I'm writing this chapter I'm surrounded by male energy: a macho husband, two sons, male gynaecologists, male doctor, male paediatrician, male social worker. My closest relative women (grandmother, mother, mother-in-law, sister-in-law) represent male energy and for that reason have a hard time embracing the actual males around them, which meant my husband was not getting the support neither. When we are not living in or with our female energy, we cannot except and receive the male energy or the male partners in our lives. The partners will be a source of conflict and inner turmoil. They are provoking us, females, to live a more whole life, a sane life, which includes our female existence. I have 9 uncles and 1 aunt spread over my two parents. It's the women that have a strong sense of female energy that were actually able to help me out over the period of potential overload, psychosis, and potential divorce. It was a first time and wonderful experience to actually have help offered and receive the emotional support for the first time in my life. At least as a mommy, but what felt to me as the very first actual time in my life I could truly have and receive guidance, support and help. Until that time I saw myself as a free, independent unit. When we see ourselves as individuals or function from that sense of freedom craving supportive mechanisms, life hits us hard when we are forced back into a sense of connectedness with others. We don't live our lives separately and we are not in control of it, even if our mind thinks we are and should be. Consciousness controls us.

Motherhood is something you do from a sense of wholeness and connectedness in this day and age, otherwise it will drive you insane. Current day parents were raised in total liberty and freedom, in general sense, and their children have become strong willed, spirited and highly developed children. Don't we all know the individuals, maybe someone else's mom, from the last generation that has gone to partial or complete frustration, depression, aloofness, isolation, anger, resentment or such? The bitter woman. Yes, and the older generations were handling two, three, four, five times the amount of children you will handle and there were no machines or services to help them out. Nothing was easy. Nothing is easy. But the bitterness and resentment within herself, the mother, as well her children (probably your parents) is existent. Nowadays, we don't want to just survive our current conditions, we want and can create our lives more consciously with an awareness about internal happiness.

We are at the same time overloaded with information and bombarded with technology and a more individualistic society. We live, current parents, with internal damage from childhood and a global society and a planet to save. The American Dream doesn't exist anymore or has long changed. Families have separated themselves from each other physically and therefor emotionally. Family life is dead, unless you revive it. The separation in the (Western) societies makes the MOM job extra challenging and the expectations in our couple's relationship make it extra challenging. How are you going to 'stick it out'? It's not taboo or impossible any more to be divorced or a single parent compared to older generations. Although for myself I felt it was quite an impossible choice and my drive to be a family was bigger than living my new life as a separated mom. On top of this individualization: there is an information overload and an access to global resources which makes us even more responsible in our minds and our choices. Previous generations were bombarded with one kind of media and led by it, current generations are a multichannel of media and feel overloaded on what to do and not to do. Where is that pot of gold going to be? The answer is as usual: from the inside. The rest of it is survival and (re)creation. Older generations were to care for primaries, like household and education, but nowadays it's not sufficient to raise your child based on primaries like feeding, dressing and schooling. We need to tender to their psychologies and happiness, which is a contradictory to the millions of over-drugged children simply for being to strong willed, intelligent and wise. We have become both the parent and the child a more complexed, intertwined and demanding individual within a more complexed, intertwined and demanding society. We don't want to be disciplined or neglected, neither the parent nor the child. Unhappiness is no longer the norm and playing on the streets and in nature, where sanity is usually found, is not so normal anymore. Moms don't want to be 100% career oriented like the ones from the 80's and 90's, neither do they want to be a stay at home mom from the 60's and 70's. It has to be something in between, but which employer or society allows that kind of work-life balance? They want a good balance between all their activities and between themselves and their children, but they feel rushed and divided. A division of time, that is not always translated into financial ends coming together or any kind of economical structure that supports the role of a mother. No wonder, Scandinavian countries have started with a year of parental leave for both fathers and mothers to raise their babies. At least to care for baby and figure things out before going back to the work force.

Compared to older generations, our secrets are not to be kept behind closed doors any longer. The so called 'dirty laundry' is now public through our own awareness of it and if not through direct means, it will probably play hide and seek, and found, through social media. Our internet has a strong force to connect and an even stronger force for individuals to be unconnected, welcome 'screen time' and negativity. Negative influences as dangers and threats of the online world including sexual harassment, bullying, media pressure, loss of self either by people you know or don't know. This online world especially dangerous, if children or yourself are not compensated and guided by 'real' life decisions which then becomes a danger to both parents and their children. Unhappy individuals, both parents and children, need follow up in order to stay on the road of fulfilment and prevent making the wrong decisions which leads them further into a negative spiral.

Today's individualistic society is slowly growing into a connected society which does not accept a lonely path towards real or spiritual death. At the moment we are overloaded with our daily work plus the daily uploading and downloading of our 'life's intelligence' programs and DNA codes into our bodies and the Matrix, whilst fighting off the negative influences. It does not work for everyone. The negative influences are big, strong and varied. It probably needs two more generations of a portion of positive people to break the bad consciousness, raising a portion of positive children to raise to the top. We, as a people, are a bit lost in this transition, but we will find our way to a more calm and composed manner if the majority wants to break through and wake up to a new world.

Even if it doesn't happen, our jobs of raising children and becoming happy people still carries on. It did for previous generations and it does for ours. Maybe we can get the most hope from that perspective: the past. They were not with less wars or less challenges and they still did an amazing job! Even if the results are not hopeful, they built a platform for us to proceed. There is your power; the people we elect, the voices unheard, the choices we make and the decisions we take. Each one of us, will lead to a bright future when we can stick with conscious, bright choices to our soul's abilities. And even if that fails and Apocalypse is falling on our heads (which in Syria it does) we still have our inner consciousness and a safe haven for our souls when we have surrendered and docked at our inner-peace haven. We might even ascend to a better realm or a better planet like ancient civilizations have done, who knows? The universe is expansive and we don't know much about it in the mainstream. This is also why it is important for you to step out of the things that were taught to you and brought you a lot of unhappiness, cravings, addictions, desperations and such. The rat race. Step out of it and start collecting information and thoughts that seem more true to you; something that could possibly be true. All beginnings are good, as long as they are not mainstream, things like aliens, demons, unicorns, fairies, witches, dragons, star seeds, collaborations, magic, alchemy, universal grids, shamanism and so on. Anything at the moment is better than being enslaved in corporate society and corporate life and a corporate body; you feel enslaved that way!

Many children's (behavioral) diseases have been created along the way of which most commonly "spread" are ADD, obesity, suicide, anorexia, allergies, autism and others. It's funny to notice that not one of these diseases are contagious or inherited. Diet, nutrition, stress, toxins and especially a sick upbringing and a sick society are at cause. It is deteriorating, killing and sickening our bodies, our DNA and our souls. These modern day diseases are a tough cookie for parents, schools and health organizations to get their grips on and to deal with. And yet, how come I ask myself? If they were doing a "better", more conscious job, wouldn't they be promoting health and happiness of the body, mind and soul? A more conscious way of living and parenting, including the governmental organizations that parent us? And what about the doctors, teachers and everyone else involved in the world of parents and children? We surely are sick if we need to drug our children into "being normal".

Distanced from our family tribe, through work and personal wishes, makes other tribes in need of assisting us and our children. Immigration does not come without cost. We are not to fall through the many gaps of the web we have woven. Society has become a web of countless gaps. Any age group will feel the pressure of one or more of the gaps in current society which we become more and more aware of as our vulnerability as an individual grows. Age, disease, poverty and racism are one such thing. White supremacy thinks it "has it all" and yet, our society is made up of individuals of age, disease and race. Where are our elders? Where are those spirited, wise people gone? What have you been hit with? Where do you need guidance? It could be addiction, boredom, no sense of direction, overworking, over-performing, meeting financial ends, technology, the internet, entrepreneurship, marriage, no marriage, appearance, fashion, health, terrorism, over-spirituality, travel, environmentalism, nutrition etc. The spectrum of choice, solutions, information and possibilities has become countless - and totally subjective - in our time and age. Try keeping your peace of mind in that web of gaps and opportunities. The trick in our day and age would be to go back to basis, basics, and more basics. This is the trend of minimalism and downsizing which works as a medicine on its own. The less we have, the less we need to worry. The closer to nature, the better we feel. We are cared for by the mother of all people Mother Nature, Gaia. My mom was right: keep it simple! The industrialization, medical industry and wars of the 40's, 50's, is taking its revenge on this generation. Convenience and consumption have taken over our sanity and sensibility. The people are creating a revolution in the minds and by going eco, bio, small business, local, animal friendly, planet friendly, people friendly, mystic, humanitarian, spiritual (by the spirit) and such. Let us go back to nature and find the Buddha within. That is the message of all. So much for industrialization and commercializing.

Being Buddha, Being Inner Peace

Why can no-one help you? And what are those skeletons in the closet? Like I said, as a wom(b)an you are not the innocent daughter or daughter-in-law anymore. You have something to prove now: being a good mother. That is what you constantly need to prove. And you will feel the effect much more and especially when you are sensitive to it. People are there to keep you focussed and point out any flaws or mistakes. This might be advice, this might be criticism, this might be guilt, this might be blame, this might be worry and this might be help. Whatever it is, it depends on the extent of the emotional drama behind the point the person is trying to make to you. Women will feel concerned about your baby, even if you don't want them to impose and perhaps that's a natural instinct and survival mechanism of living in tribes. In most cases, the intention is not from a positive attitude when you receive yet another batch of critics, surely it will bring a lot of frustration to the table from either you or the other. That too will pass. For the most part. When you have earned your years and when you don't mind a good piece of comparison or advice, you can start seeing the bigger picture of your role as a mother and not take it as personal. Whatever people say on a personal note to you, even if it is your children, says most about themselves and has a gift for you to take away. When you are seeking a break of current patterns and a next step on enlightenment, you can ask yourself: what if they are right? What if I am a witch? What if I'm a magician? What if I am what they say? So what?

You might have already experienced these kind of conflicts and drama when you got engaged or certainly during marriage preparations and celebrations. You might have contributed a big part of the drama: bridezilla. You are by default more involved in becoming a wife or a mother, more than you wish you were or had intended.

Consider "Being Buddha" to pass by in life. Buddha once, doesn't mean that you can hold on to it all the time, especially in the beginning of your Buddha journey. You might hit a period where it all hits you again, especially if you tend to hold your emotions or went too male or too feminine in your activities and energies for an extensive time. This is where the moon cycles and astrological calendar bring about a chunk of awareness. Not one day is the same. Every day has a different potential and guidance, just like the moon fading in and out, your energies are fading in and out. These tools are an excellent way of self-discovery and assertiveness when direct access or communication of your feelings is not your strongest asset (yet). Talking doesn't mean you are in touch with your core self or your feelings. Being inwards also does not mean that you know yourself yet and how to direct your being and talents. All of the natural medicine and tools you can use or feel attracted to in the slightest sense, will reinforce your life purpose.

During the hectic motherhood I was inclined to make a dreamcatcher, than a friend actually made a beautiful one without me knowing about it and once she finished, we held a small workshop with other women about setting your intentions for a dreamcatcher. I managed to continue the process by following whatever came up for me and the intention that came to me is wanting to be more in touch with my feminine energy and subsequently the mystic life.

The dreamcatcher took a lot of symbolic, unconscious, meanings in the process of making it. Breaking patterns, breaking old karma, breaking the ties I have with those things that don't suit me, even with society at large; all the heritage so to speak. Usually these things can involve some screaming to break it loose from the body and other times it is a silent allowance or forgiveness. Unraveling, unlearning and undoing ourselves is the most important process of living a meaningful life. And you will be surprised how much we suppress! Getting to a point of making this your biggest past time is a tremendous effort of letting go, opening up, allowing yourself, not feeling guilty (mom guilt included!). Taking those baby steps to self-care and self-expression are tremendous. Now we remember, or we can allow ourselves to remember, how vulnerable our babies feel and how we must have felt when we were those tiny bodies making huge steps in life. My heart goes out to them. Self-care, self-love and self-expression are the most important work you can do yourself and for your children. And I'm telling and reminding myself of course to not stay on status quo. It's not because I've achieved so much from a ground 0 or from the pit of -10 I get to be fulfilled by all means, no there are areas I want to discover more, there are activities I want to do, there are commitments I want to follow up on, there are emotions in the 10+ range I want to experience, there are relationships I want to encounter, there is support I want to receive. Your activities for self-care, self-love and self-expression are all inclusive, including the shopping, groceries, cooking, eating, feeding, dressing up, bathing, nourishing, fitness, activities, intellect and so on which are or are supposed to be daily motions of life running through us. The more we can open up to these activities as a self-love, self-care and self-expression method, the more we become ourselves and find the strength of the universe instead of letting these things run us down in lack, poverty and disease.

Even if you are not doing this out of self, you are still doing it out of self. But you are doing it out of a ground 0 or a lack of self. Like the native cultures, everything is sacred, everything has meaning, every gesture is intentional or through intention. Look how gorgeous they make themselves, full of encouraging symbols, full of stories, full of intentions, full of power, full of connections and so on. Why are we - Westerners - not meant to live that way? On a side note: I'm not saying again that things are perfect or done a 100% of the time. Of course I will still eat a pizza, wear ugly sneakers, knock my head and use the occasional F-word conversation. We don't live excluded from our Western pop culture and we don't need to reject it 100% in order to live a life of self-respect, although unfortunately there is a bare minimum of self-respect in pop-culture. If there is any? Breaking free of society's mind control or should I say 'mind fuck' is becoming Wild. The growing community of wild women and men is becoming stronger with the day.

Unleashing your creative, social side

The things you can do while your baby is awake and with you, do them while your baby is awake and with you. The things that are really "you time" keep them for the nap or night time (of your baby). So in other words: don't do household things during your baby's nap time. Even if they need to be done, your baby's nap time probably doesn't last that long especially with an (inter)active baby. This kind of baby and any baby for that matter will demand all your attention and reactiveness in order to develop his active brain, in particular the first 6-7 months.

In month 7-9 the baby their intelligent brain will start to learn to play on it's own and this will give you back your hands and time a little. My second son was a sleepy baby and never demanded as much interaction as the "brainy" first one. The second prefers physical touch, practical jokes and is a social butterfly. It seems that second babies are more easy-going. Every baby is different and demands a different side of you. It is this relationship that starts from the start. The better you know your baby, the better you know the potentials in yourself and what side of yourself you are exploring. Your children are karmic incarnations of you.

When this part is left neglected, ignored, shamed or blamed you will damn yourself along the way, and stay stuck on ground 0. Your children will grow up insanely, meaning half, instead of sane (whole person). To me, this along with practical care taking, is a reason I would prefer lesser children. Even one. There is too much to handle for my hands and my brain. I guess, as time passes and the heart grows, there is more space for more children. I try to imagine having three or a girl, but it is just too much for one mother and father I wonder.

While baby is with you, you can listen to a Podcast, Tedtalk, Audiobook or such. Consider activities like taking a shower, getting dressed, doing make-up whilst your baby is with you. And these moments is when you can listen to background music or talks. The "you time" when you are alone and concentrated would be things like:

- checking emails
- admin
- surfing the net
- working on the laptop
- reading a book
- writing a book
- drawing, creating or other creativeness
- journaling
- meditation, yoga

- watching a series, documentary or movie even in daytime
- connecting with people
- working on your projects!

As a mommy, and especially as a creative "fulltime" mommy a.k.a. stay at home mommy, you will come up with new ideas, projects and potential businesses. Obviously they would involve babies, children or such. None of it necessarily, but likely. You will see the gaps in your world of having a baby, the society, the neighborhood you live in, the stuff you use, the innovations, future projections. So this is your chance for changing around your career and working on a meaningful future. Is that not what so many people dream of doing? Opening up their own business? Working flexible hours? More involvement with their families? Needless to say that having your own business, big, small or tiny requires constant care. So you are basically having a 2nd (3rd, 4th, 5th..) baby, besides your husband, pet and house. However, you don't need to "think big". The act and the process of doing something you like, something meaningful and something you are dedicating your "you time" to is meaningful in itself, whatever the outcome. This can be a coffee or tea ritual only.

If you can contribute to your own or someone else's life, even if they are your children or the collective consciousness, than I suppose it is as rewarding as making it into something in exchange for money. You might find yourself exchanging goods or services, doing voluntary work, crafting, donating or selling your second hand things. Or writing about your experience! This involvement and commitment is the reason I'm writing this book. And believe me, the nap are no more than 30 minutes! Most of this is written at night, early mornings and during editing phase every little minute in between or sitting beside them at their bath.

Your mother is your example

My mom was a great example of a creative "stay at home" mom. When I was around 10 years old (my youngest sibling was 2 years old) she set up a crafty play group for children age 7-14 years and named it "Itchy Fingers". She received the children at a friend's place in the open air and taught them a new crafty activity. She also was teaching aerobics in a local gym after she had followed years of aerobics herself. When she went back to the job market, at the age of 40+, she went back to her very original profession as a computer science engineer from 10 years previous. After pension, and following my dad's career, she restarted her career again at the engineering job. It seems that we are only, or mostly, proud of our moms when they do things for themselves, creatively or for their career. Especially after the Early Childhood Years I would say.

I have an eight years younger brother and a four years younger sister. Later when all her kids moved out, around her pension time, she took on the crafty activities and specialized in "fabric paintings". She gives workshops and helps orphanage children, and is known in Singapore as an artist. She aspires to study for being a certified Art Therapist.

My mom made motherhood look easy. She cooked a fresh meal every single day of the week and she is still doing that for my dad after 33 years. We hardly or never had take-in. We ate at a Chinese restaurant maybe once per year. Alright, in Singapore she had more of a break because it was more practical and cost effective to eat at the farmer's foodcourt. She was there for lunch time during the school's lunch break. In The Netherlands no lunches or break times are provided at school. She cleaned the house herself and took care of the three of us and our father. She never complained one day. Alright, maybe one. She's very pragmatic in that sense. She also kept our photo books, journaled our lives and promoted our spirit to be independent, successful and especially "free" human beings.

I might not have felt encouraged and supported in my alternative view to life. Especially after my continuous burn outs and toxic boyfriends, I started to fail from the inside. My sense of success and freedom were failing me hard. I was trying to copy the success of my self made parents. Both my parents had successful careers, as a treasury director and computer engineer, with no master or university degree in their pocket. So me, somehow, had more ambition to find an employee during my studies rather than focus on a my studies for the time being. Their example of a solid marriage and moving countries to see the world, was also my ideal. I failed miserably. I failed at all of it. At least, from an inner happiness and health perspective.

My career or talents never were appreciated by anyone and never picked up at any given time, and I was not particularly affirming myself with one sense of career or direction in my mind. I did not work in the big enterprises with the right infrastructure until my thirties. It was a fertile soil for being my own liberated person, but along with constant sense of "loss".

My intimate life remained toxic despite all the coaches I had seen. Moving countries came at a big cost and it was the only thing I was good at. So far, into marriage, things seemed just perfect from the outside. It was a "fatamorgana"; from reality nothing was matching up from the inside. I had no degree, no CV, no career, no support, no finance and a lot of instability within because I had never known to live a stable or solid life. By the time I was born a mother, it came crumbling down on my head an I remained with one thing: it was my child. My newborn Raphael, archangel of healing. And that is what the dear angel brought me. A whole lot of healing, more than any coach or therapist could possibly give me. I needed my firstborn to bring me so much healing in order to rise again out of the ashes, like the Phoenix. This depiction might show you on some level that we don't need something to start out life with, our life will live itself anyway. If we were given minimal gifts or only certain gifts, the other gifts are still there but we need to seek for them a little harder than another. And our initial gifts are different. We all have unique stories and yet, so many of them come to the same road of loneliness and suffering, no matter how much you had or did not have. Either you get the master degree and feel miserable in your career or you didn't go to school and feel miserable. Either you were smothered in love and feel miserable or you were loved less and feel miserable. Either you were grown up to be independent and free and you feel miserable or you were kept at close ties and still feel miserable.

We cannot rewrite the actual past, but we can rewrite it in our memories, and rewire our brains, filter out the subconsciousness of toxicity. There is a lot we can do about it, in each and every moment and with awareness it becomes easier to actually work on the actual work of releasing, forgiving, letting go, cutting cords, and healing the wounds

Creating your tribe

When you cannot depend on your family for whatever reason, and clearly when you live far from family, you will want to create your own tribe. This tribe is made of friends and of people that are like friends, but that want to support you and vice versa in times of need and support and company. You can ask each other to help out with rides to nursery, make meals, hold the children after nursery or school, babysit on a date night, do playdates, go to the park, hold coffee mornings and so on. You should realize that you don't have your usual tribe and tribal activities: your family members neither your long term friends from back home or where you initially grew up.

Another term for tribe is Framily. The Urban Dictionary describes a tribe as Framily: when friends become like family, they're framily, closer than close, they may know you better than your own family. Or rather (this is a different definition): a group of friends, who are close like family. In the best case your tribe or framily members know each other as well. That way you can have a group dynamism. Framily members don't necessarily need to have children! In some cases, it's more convenient and they might be more close to you, if they don't have the kiddos! Listen: "having the kiddos" sounds reliable. The worry and care over their own children is that what keeps parents apart, so having members out there with more availability, energy and care and fun factor for your family is just awesome. These kind of uncles and aunts, non-parents, can be especially valuable to your child, even more so at a later age. We have lost a tribal living in modern day society, more so with migrated families and we will continue to seek it.

When your child is older (s)he can spend quality time or quality talks in order to share with someone other than their own parents their upbringing, even to vent and get advice. The role of such an official or unofficial godmother or godfather becomes important in certain phases of your child's development. If they don't find these trustworthy individuals of age, they are more likely to find them among older peers or strangers, even if they are of bad influence. They might not have the best agenda or best intentions with your youngster, even downright dangerous intentions.

The same replacement of "something lost within the family" can happen when the father role of the actual father is absent, neglected or not so present. The child, even as an adult, will keep on seeking for a father-like type that will replace the missing bond and experience as a child. A more healthy approach is to facilitate the absent role by interaction and celebrations with uncles. I mention celebrations, because if the father is absent, your child will still want a father-like type to encourage and applaud for the milestones and personal achievements in their life. Especially for boys, there is an phase in the age of 6-10 years, where the boy needs more than just one father to look up to. The book 'Raising boys' talk about his phase and we become more familiar with the importance of becoming a man when we study the initiation of manhood.

In modern day life we "lost something" and it is big. We lost the manhood which is surrounded by brotherhood as well as the motherhood which is surrounded by sisterhood. And now we are trying to find it back through almost artificial means. The good thing is that becoming and being aware of this part of culture and society, can help you to calm down and be somewhat OK with this part of culture. Also, would you like to live in a community? Or would you need some part-time community, live with a fixed community part-time or only live communal during a certain season? These are valid questions to ponder. I know friends that moved countries and set up their own tiny community very consciously and I see possibilities of finding the right balance of community with your own online or offline tribe. It needs some figuring out and putting together the puzzle pieces to get it finalized and into action, because finances and responsibilities usually play big parts in what we see as possible and impossible. We live in a world of abundance. There is enough for everyone. Nature does not discriminate: she provides everyone willingly with food if evenly grown or distributed. So instead of impossible, we need in our own lives to think I'M-possible to make the smaller and bigger changes that can lead to better happiness and health. This was the only reason I and my husband got to move houses or countries on our own initiative. We dared it possible, despite losing jobs.

I would also like to mention that there are many secrets to be found with ancient civilizations, native cultures and the current day tribes. Tribes don't experience the anxious, neurotic mothers and crying babies. The tribal living explains a lot about the problems we encounter in modern day society and individualist family life. We can gain wisdom, tips, tricks and a whole lot of consciousness from these old cultures.

Self-support, Self-care and Self-love

You will need to find your ways and means in order to support your own self in this new mom job. With the years, you become more experienced, more skilled, more supported. You will create a network with other colleagues and associates, including professionals, that you can "exploit" in a positive way. Meaning: take the advantage of what professionals can do for you as a mother. It is your first time and it is not their first time. Often, I believe, help is offered to a mom and she will not take it. We are too full of ego in the beginning because "we should do it all" and it is considered normal "to do it all". That was the example we had over the generations of "femininity".

How awfully wrong. Outright disgusting if you ask me. Feminism is about "doing it all"? So now us women are supposed to become men and some super creature? Grow some balls and perhaps a tail? Somehow in getting careers as women, we should have thought ourselves of a balance of the working hours and the respect for our true femininity. I'm shouting from the rooftops and into my own ears: the age of individuality is over, help each other! Jump on the opportunity! Delegate tasks! Get a Cleaning Lady! get an Au Pair! Get over yourself first and foremost. Being and becoming the woman you are, supported and intertwined, won't make you less of a super woman. Doing less and being more will. Both housework and outside jobs are overrated, especially for women. We can do it all, yes, we can do one really good, yes, we can do both really well, yes, but at the end of the day: who really cares and gives a f*.

If you are still feeling insane, not whole, then you are not in your whole. The whole of being and feeling whole and doing wholeness things wholeheartedly and as a whoman or wombman or simply a SHE. Not the "hole" as in your hole and up their hole. Why do we even want to go there? Because we have "lost something" and we've lost it really very well. It has been a war of the men v.s. the women. This subject is another book on its own. Just the awareness that the product you are today, be it either a man, a woman or something else has a full history of tied up stories, stigmas, paradigms and dark secrets which reside for bigger parts with the churches, Vatican and other politics. It is time to unravel that smelly cellar of the Vatican and come out with the truth of men and women.

Was woman really created from the men's rib? Or was it from the woman's womb? Was Jesus really single or was he married with children? Was it not Mary Magdalene who was as much of a master and valued as Jesus was? Whatever the answers to universal questions, it is up to you to seek your truth, your tribe and create the life style that best fits your internal happiness and (mental) health.

Have you thought about Life Coaching? Have you done something differently lately? Let's first look at some essentials to make life a little lighter than it is right now.

Mommy's and Baby's Essentials (List of Tips)

These items were essential for my survival. They also make a great "At Home" gift for the new mommy.

- Casio Illuminator, Baby G, sports-watch or a Smartwatch. I personally adore the Pebble and it works with my Android phone (as well as IOS). Although like any gadget, you have to get into it. Otherwise; a watch with small internal light to read the time in the dark. The watches with the fluorescent indicators will not last you through the whole night. The fluorescent that lasted all night was made of a toxic ingredient which is banned now.

- Double walled glasses for tea, coffee, cold drinks and a travel thermo for on the road. You'll make your drink but won't get to it in an hour or so. It's nice to come back to your hot or cold drink and still find it in a good or excellent temperature.

- Apps to track your health and lack of hours of sleep if you wish to do so. You might consider a smartwatch.

- Google assistance on your phone with a speaker in each important room to help look up things, plan and communicate hands-free.

- A contact list of recommended clinics and hospitals for you and your infant, for all the cases you want to drop by quickly. Consider subscribing yourself at the hospitals you might be visiting to skip registration process.

- Sneakers and slip-on shoes. The slip on shoes are also necessary during the pregnancy, when the belly gets in the way of you and your feet.

- A bathrobe as a towel for after the shower to dry up and move quickly. And another bathrobe that makes you feel good to present yourself at the door when the bell rings or when you have visitors to cover your pj.

- Some small purse to carry your phone, house keys, payment card and a pacifier which you carry with you all of the time in order not to leave your purse or belongings behind or have them stolen. I love the durability and class of Furla.

- Good protection case for the phone and to strap it on the arms or waist. And a phone holder or speaker for in the car.

- Baby carrier or sling, or both. The sling is used during the newborn phase, but some carriers also start from month 1.

- Breastfeeding t-shirt and cover up cloth for breastfeeding in public, popular or luxury places. Cloth hair bands to keep your hair out of your face.

- A powerful alternative to coffee like powdered tea, matcha tea, and powerful snacks like protein bars. As well as Magnesium, Calcium and Vitamin C tablets that dissolve in water.

- Essential oils, whatever they are, you can find a good use for them. Do not underestimate the power of aromatherapy, cleaning, cleansing, healing, vibrating on higher levels, introducing new frequencies and so forth with the help of essential oils.

- Calming aromatherapy and a calming, herbal tincture like Dr. Bach or others to change your mood, wake you up or help you when nervous.

- Bath essential salts and magnesium.

- Self care kit of organic creams, makeup etc for a sensitive body. Parfum-free perfume and aluminium-free deodorant. BPA-free shampoo for mom and baby. Use the organic products you would use for your baby so you can take a bath together.

- Subscription to a mommy/parent or other magazine to look forward to receiving.

- Monthly subscription for a massage and a beauty salon.

- Coffee presser to make your cup of goodness or a machine to work on those caffeine shots! Of course, whilst breastfeeding, there will be less drinking coffees but then there will be a time where you'll need your coffee to stay awake.

- Monthly (or weekly!) foot massage and any other type of massage, facial, manicure and pedicure treatments.

Baby's Sleep Essentials

- 2 sets of blankets, if one being washed, to lie down on one and be covered by the second. Also when baby is curled up on the blanket, you can cover the baby with the 2nd blanket.

- Musical soft toy, so you can put the music close to baby, take it with you outdoor and alternate it if you have another musical instrument attached to the bed. Start playing this music whilst baby is in the belly so baby will recognize this as a familiar and soothing sound.

- Baby husher machine, app or recording that gives shushes or white noise. It could be nature sounds instead of hushing or white noise. The hush machine or a recording on a recording device is most preferred, not your phone - a phone receives calls, radiates and is a general disturbance - and not a hairdryer, because it is a danger if you fall asleep or drop it on baby. White noise can alternatively be from the stove top where you carry your baby in a carrier.

Why hiring a consultant is a shortcut

Consultants or experts are hired because of their expertise in a given area. A consultant has expertise, a mentor has experience. A mentor is ahead of you and will guide you to the secrets and shortcuts of whatever you are mentored on. They will also give you hints on how you are performing. A consultant or expert is no luxury during your entire postpartum experience, motherhood and parenthood.

We don't learn to be a parent, be a mother, take care of a baby or parent our children. Besides, as a parent you are constantly confronted with life itself and the limitations and opportunities within that framework, which is absolutely challenging.

Would you give it a try to work on yourself, your stories, your questions, your desires, wishes and goals? And you are going to make your move to experience some therapy or seek help? How to understand the difference between a psychiatrist, psychology, coach, therapist, mentor and counsellor? And when to use which therapist?

Different options for seeking help

Counsellors have specialized training in such things as healthy communication, parenting, social skills, career development skills, and mental and emotional or psychological underlying motivations and reasoning. They focus on dysfunctions and shortcomings in order to catchup with a wishful pace, speed or situation. A social worker can be trained as a counsellor. Therapists have such skills but are more specialized in a certain technique.

A person in need of healing or with too many troubles, like addictions or a weakened spirit, is not yet ready for coaching and should be referred to a counsellor and therapist.

A coach is goal oriented and has a cheerleading attitude. Coaches originate from the sports; a sports coach and fitness coach. The diet coach and career coach is widely accepted. In the mental, emotional, spiritual arena they do not necessarily require expertise or experience, but they will relate through their own life's evolution and empathy. Coaches help you to clarify your wants and needs, your creations, your passion and your skills and transformations in order to be a better version of yourself. Coaching can be ultimately healing. A coach does not make decisions for you, they facilitate for you to make decisions yourself that are empowering and lead you towards your goals. Also, it is very likely that breakthroughs in one area of self-care, will reflect on all other parts of your life like a chain reaction. Nothing is more empowering and healing than becoming the you you were meant to be all along the way.

Why is coaching popular and how does it help?

A coach, including pregnancy and birth coaches or doulas, sounds less intimidating than a psychologist or therapist. When we feel good about ourselves and our life, we might want to go to the next level of achievement or a quicker route to our goals by seeking a coach. A sportsperson will never do sports without his or her coach(es)! As a great business man will always hire experts and coaches. The great thing about coaches is that they listen and provoke. They do not accept any bullshit and they keep you in your power. They want the best of you. In order to get you ahead, they ask you questions and cheer you on.

Dreams and Desires need to be supported

I have experience with coaches, therapists and with counsellors, psychologists and psychiatrists. A therapist or psychiatrist might have a coaching background and, most importantly, attitude and a coach might have a attitude of a healer or therapist. Perhaps it is more important to look at the attitude of the professional you are seeking, for, rather than their exact title or technique. A coach is objective, clear, all ears, non-judgemental, knowledgeable, motivating, inspires and will ask you questions, for you to hear yourself.

When to see a counsellor or therapist and when to see a coach?

"Counseling primarily deals with the past to the present. Coaching primarily deals with the present to the future.

Counseling is more about processing and healing, coaching is more about envisioning and growing. So depending on what you feel the most, the burden or the passion at this very moment, will show if you need to work on the past or on the future. Is the past holding you back? Or is the future a question mark for you? Also, when we have worked on our past and find ourselves at peace or even in total chaos, we can ask a coach to give us the push forward and to work on our dreams and desires, even when they are still unknown and residing in the dark.

There are counsellors that inhibit both therapy and coaching. So look for the person that 'speaks' to you and remain respectful of your own experience. If you don't enjoy the therapy or coaching relationship, then move on to the next. It's up to you to go once or several times or for a more frequent visit.

Welcome on board,

Welcome to the Mothership; the vessel of life.

- Andromeda L.C.

7 Peace on Earth Comes with a Peaceful Birth

This chapter talks about breastfeeding failures (BFF), Post Partum Depressions (PPD) and Birth Violations (BV). I would like to start out by talking about the breastfeeding and the failures of achieving a consistent breastfeeding and the feelings that comes with this experience.

How much milk to feed your baby

Breast milk is typically produced on demand. Baby's suckling of the nipples signals to the mama's body that it needs milk and more milk to come. It is an indication of keeping the milk supply ongoing, because as long as the nipples are suckled, milk will be on demand for years to come. Even without suckling the breasts are ready to restart the production for years to come. The less baby nurses, the less mama's body makes milk. As long as your baby is feeding of a breast, there is milk, there is in my opinion no real worry about the amount of milk provided or taken by your baby, because it's an intuitive process and baby knows how much to drink or not to drink. Even the mother's body knows which kind of milk to produce for her baby in that particular time.

Suckling tends to lead to cloves and, cloves lead to bleeding and infections or bacteria entering the wounds, which leads to Mastitis. You might want to restrain the feeding to 45-50 minutes per breast to not overstimulate and prevent soar nipples. I will dedicate a whole section to treating and healing Mastitis from my personal experience with healing this very common condition, both in the hospital and at home.

Breast and bottle simultaneously is possible

A different action of the tongue is required for either breastfeeding or bottle feeding. While breastfeeding, baby's tongue goes underneath and draws nipple and milk into himself. With a bottle, baby's must stop and release the flow of milk somehow with his mouth, tongue or throat. This can lead to confusion for some babies who receive both breast and bottle, but you cannot tell if it will or will not. My second baby took breastmilk and formula milk from day 1. If he was hungry he took only formula milk, if he was thirsty he took only breastmilk. This lasted for one year. My first baby took only formula milk due to wrong latching and mastitis.

Health and bonding benefits of breastfeeding

Breastfeeding offers extensive health benefits, so consider staying with breastfeeding until the baby decides to downsize on the feeding. Breastfeeding is also extremely inexpensive and practical opposed to buying formula every 3-4 days. The budget you save can be spent on your personal care, like manicures, massages and whatever you will need to keep on the good work. You need to set a budget for this before giving birth.

Research shows a good connection between academic results and boys that are breastfed for 6 months or longer. We should be aware of the complex, nutritious, valuable milk that our bodies produce for the baby and how it can replace a cow milk formula if we need the formula. It is a miraculous superpower and keeps adjusting the substance to the needs of your particular baby. A formula will not do that, yet it will grow up your baby as sufficient as the breastfed baby. I have an example of both, my first baby was breastfed for only one month, the second one took breast and bottle for one year. They are equally healthy, happy and intelligent, although the second boy was and is much more of a mommy's boy.

Another scientific benefit for the mother is that she will lower her risk of all sorts of disease like cancers, arthritis and Alzheimer for every month extra breastfed.

Breastfeeding Dads

Breastfeeding offers a way for the Dad to be involved and bond with baby and you! Instead of him offering a bottle to baby, he can sit with you at a breastfeeding session and stay seated while he offers you a tea and a talk. He can also sit behind you, giving you back support and a welcome hug and connection. It's very intimate and I've honestly never ever done it and learnt about this option only after breastfeeding had stopped. If you consider doing it, I believe it is a great bonding moment and it will offer the dad a lot of comfort and respect in his supportive role. Dads can have a tendency to not be alienated, not supportive, when their self-esteem is low or when they were hurt by their past relationships, including their own mother. In fact, a man's natural instinct is to be the provider, the hunter, the protector, the supporter. So it is in his favour to share these kind of intimate moments with baby. It is also in your family unit's favour of building up a bond. A dad can be warded from a baby by his instinct or self-esteem because the baby is too fragile for him, but he won't usually have this feeling towards you, although I do not exclude anything because I have been through all the arena of negative connotations. This family unit position, which can include siblings, for a breastfeeding sessions means everyone can have best of both worlds and it can give mom a very welcome break from solitude and moment of connection with the other members. This position between mom and dad or siblings is not restricted to breastfeeding, it is also possible with bottle-feeding, of course!

Not your cup of tea
Breastfeeding should be a natural thing according to nature, yet somehow the experience feels as the most unnatural option to the majority of women. It takes practice, insights, bonding and experience and a whole lot of pain and patience. It also "sucks the life out of you" and it's a constant practice, because baby needs your breasts every 2,5 hours. It leads to all kinds of feelings of anxiety, desperation and failure.

No matter if we breastfeed or if we don't, it causes an experience of failure or guilt. It remains a complex ordeal and to the majority of women it becomes a traumatic one, especially with the first baby. We want the best for our baby, so the question that runs through our motherly system is; can we achieve and perform? The truth is that a baby needs to be fed and both ways are good, or great: breastfed, bottle or both during any which duration.

Breastfeeding toddlers and children
If you persist or continue breastfeeding, it can lead up to any age! Lots of women are breastfeeding up to 1 - 4 years of age. So, even when we think that we shouldn't be breastfeeding for no more than 1-6 months, it holds no logic according to the nature of your body. The milk keeps coming and coming. The baby and the mother will decide on the right timing to stop.

The PPD Talks
Both breastfeeding and not breastfeeding can lead to (slight or full on) depression or feelings of failure, which relate to Post Partum Depression (PPD). I believe personal-

ly, that ANY birth leads to an intensive depression of 6 months on average until the body has made a semi-recovery and the mother and child are physically less dependant on each other. After the initial 6 months the depression will mellow down and come in phases of physical pain which a height at 11-12 months of age. After the First Birthday, everything will seem to go much better and there will be new challenges.

As a matter of fact, we cannot really know if the breastfeeding is helping your body to be less depressed and more at ease or if your psyche feels depressed being the absolute constant food source to your baby. I've experienced the possibility of feeding my second baby with both breast and bottle simultaneously, according to his demand, and I think it was the perfect balance for a mother to keep her sanity. If it is possible for you and your baby to vary some breastfeeding with a bottle of breast pumped milk or with formula, that is a way to go to get your break. Personally I did not have that break with neither of my babies and I do not think I did well. Other people should be feeding your baby with bottles so you can get a rest from the routine and catch up on sleep. So, by default you will need an electric breast pump machine in order to ease out on some feeding session and perhaps asking for Daddy to stay home and going for that girl's night out or alone time.

Birth events, PPD talk and becoming unpregnant

A post-partum situation, or depression, is the situation we find ourselves in after birth up to months and years to come. The details and intensity, depend on the intensity or complexity of your birthing and healing process, including the hard work and overwhelming experience of the first year with baby. I believe, as mentioned, that ALL women have PPD for a period, more intensely in the first six months, due to the physical and psychological impact of the birth event on the body, mind and soul, as well as the aftermath and the newborn phase. Becoming unpregnant, caring for newborn, body rebalancing, body recovery, hormonal cocktails, being underfed and sleep deprived amongst other complications are not to be taken lightly. Unfortunately, society and our individual lifestyles provides no mercy.

Something can go wrong through the process of birthing and honestly, I would say; usually it does go off track somehow. The birth has affected us as a person, a new mother, a woman and in relationship to our child, as well as the world. If we cannot find an inner modus operandi, we can live a life of regret, trauma, sorrow and sadness.

I believe PPD comes in various degrees. Post Partum Depression can also exist for years, and years, and years, to come in the mother's world and the mother's reality. The depression can relate to any aspect of the birth, the people surrounding her birth, her body, the baby's, the child as a person or her own life as a mother.

A new way of looking at pregnancy and beyond

Ideally the mother will bond with her baby despite the depression. Any mother can find herself, over the years, in a situation where she rejects the baby, either emotionally or psychically. This does not happen by a conscious decision, rather it happens by a physical dislike and incapability of bonding and caring, for the baby or the person for a certain hour, day, week, month or year. It is stronger than herself. The other possibility is for her to have the will to take care of her baby, yet finding herself blocked and incapable to take the actual actions and set in a caretaker's role and behavior. I know and believe this experience can also come later on in motherhood. In that sense, there is an amazing chemistry and force at play when it comes to mothers, fathers and their children continuing a life of unity.

I'm a believer that the old concept of Post Partum Depression is not the right narrative for what PPD actually insinuates. We all are depressed, suppressed, oppressed and what not in various degrees on various levels. How about we call it Post Party Depression? Life a hangover, our body needs to get out of the rush from a late night. The only difference, that the party of birthing continues for over a year and the hangover is continues. A birth of a mother and the raising of a child, will bring out the best in us, but only if we allow to evolve with the change. Becoming parents, coming of age and entering new decades in our lives has an extreme significant meaning. To great sadness we have lost all the native tales, rituals, passings, meaning and symbolism that go along with these rites of passages. We are lost in a limbo land when it comes down to Western cultures and American Pop culture.

PPD narrated solely as an extreme possibility of depression or neglect of the baby, is not the correct depiction of what might happen after birth or the fear of it. It is much more personal than that and yes, there will and is certainly an effect postpartum. Life does not stop at the birth event. I am a firm believer, from a biological and practical point of view, that ALL mothers go through 9-18 months of becoming unpregnant, which is to be considered as part of the 9-10 months of pregnancy. Becoming unpregnant can last for at least 1,5 year postpartum and suffer from a period of depression for any one reason, situation, relationship or interaction before, since or beyond the birth event. Breastfeeding, sleep deprivation, lack of nutrition, change of lifestyle, becoming a family, new hierarchy and relationships, loss of work, loss of income, loss of freedom and flexibility are all reasons for a mother to become sad, angry or depressed. There is, as previously mentioned, a physical change which impacts the persona more than the pregnancy might have effected the mother: physical tiredness, an isolated bubble, increased pregnancy brain, a new chemistry balance, a hormonal cleansing, new breasts and body, but also life, marriage, groceries, getting dressed, hygiene, schedules and so much more.

Becoming unpregnant in the year after birth and the direct recovery in the months after birth are underestimated. We are not pregnant 9 months, neither 12. We are pregnant for at least 24 months until the baby has had his first birthday. It is a beautiful period with a lot of depression, but also inspiration and aspiration. We keep on birthing ourselves and our concepts into the world. Perhaps, we are forever pregnant as Mothers. We carry the World in our Womb.

The wounding of Mothers

A mother does not feel like a mother directly at birth of her child. Nature will play its forces, yet it takes time, dedication and especially self-confidence to own the title of mother. Perhaps it does come more as a title, despite the holistic change the woman passes through with the birth event, the relationship with her child can be effected or not by many other reasons, which makes her less of a mother. The relationship with her child can be affected for the rest of their lives. I've seen this experience in my own family system, and probably every family has babies that were disowned or not included. I think some mothers never exit the depression and they will never be (self) diagnosed for it. It's an extremely hard reality for women to detect or admit that they did not really want to be a mother or could not accept their child, physically or spiritually. Acceptance of the negative truth, sets us free and can bring positive change. Accepting and shouting out the negative truths, even if you do not agree or feel them, is liberating: yes, I'm depressed! yes, I'm hurt! yes, I hate this life! yes, I hate you! yes, I don't want this! yes, I feel the pain of all women! This is a revelation in itself.

At some points in motherhood you might start shouting out your sorrows of your system and it is wonderful if it can happen. It will set more women free. You are not the only one and you are not alone. You are talking for generations of women and mothers, misunderstood and suppressed. Karma is transformed by releasing it. This is how we heal ourselves, our children and the world. This is the Mother Wound. That wound is what we carry in each one of us. man and women alike.

The secret of Motherhood

Only they will know, the mothers. A well kept secret. And the big pitfall of birthing a child, either consciously or unconsciously lives through their minds, hearts and bodies. No woman can predict how much she will be affected by birth trauma, PPD and bonding capabilities. I can only say: it WILL happen, even with the most fantastic birth, due to the psychical situation, recovery and insomnia after birth. Let us not forget the insomnia. It took me a long time to accept that THIS is the situation of all women post-partum: PPD. Even if I felt like I didn't have postpartum effects at all, especially PPD, I could not have gone by my birth unaffected. There was a birth trauma at place. And I needed recovery of both the psychical and the psychological aspects. The mind, the body, the womb and the breasts live on a different level of human, even more so when we are becoming unpregnant. The trauma lived in my being every single day, until one day I was healed for the majority by seeing professional help. I advocate for more acknowledgement and support of anyone's postpartum life. If someone disagrees with me on any of the above or if I have insulted anyones experience or birthing process, you are welcome to contact me and I will happily receive and respond to your expressions.

Birth Violation

At my mid-term echo with a specialized doctor the doctor was moving around and shaking my tummy with such a temper, I was literally shocked. I was shocked again when it continued and I didn't have the power to actually say: stop. I wanted her to stop being that rough with my tummy and baby, but I didn't feel confident enough to tell her. I suffered partly from the 'nice girl' syndrome and partly from a 'doctor is right' syndrome. She was the surgeon specialist and had to do what had to be done, right? And to make things worse, she couldn't measure or assess the requirements because the baby was sleeping. She had to keep pushing and moving again and again. This made her push and shake even more. I felt violated and then disappointed not having the necessary results of the echograph. I felt rage. I wouldn't call it "rape" but online, you can find the term "birth rape". If you consider that you might have been 'birth raped', I encourage you to seek it out in the online world of birth violation and talk to a professional or process it by other means until you feel understood.

I imagine these experiences exist even in hospital and medical experiences, other than birth. I have no firsthand information on these experiences, again you are welcome to contact me if you would like to share your story. Acknowledging what you have been through, without rationalizing it, is the first step to healing. When tools or fingers are inserted in the vagina (or anus) by the doctor or assistant, even of your baby, we can experience this as a rape. It does not need to be your most private parts, in my case it was my pregnant belly. Even when their is a medical context and without any agenda or intention of doing harm to you or your baby, it is about your experience.

There are women traumatized from Birth Rape. After I made a complaint at my own gynaecologist about the roughness and the unsuccessful assessment, he had another colleague redo the exam. It was sufficient for me to process and forget what had happened previously.

A society of intrusion

Invading and crossing decent boundaries is a violation. Wherever and whenever and with whomever it happens. As a matter of fact, as parents we can be extremely intrusive towards our children and their bodies. This is an extremely important realization within your role as an adult. Keep in mind that this is HIS or HER body and not by any means your property for you to touch, push around, pick-up, put down or whatever is necessary or unnecessary by the means of touch. Always, always ask for permission, as you are the extension to their physical capabilities and incapabilities. Never touch their private parts unless for putting a medication and in that case you ask first, like a doctor or nurse would or should do. Their private parts are theirs and theirs to keep. This is a very important protection for them consciously and unconsciously to protect them from predators or harm, even as a grown up. Imagine you were touched every day on your private parts, wether for cleaning or potty training, and that feeling of being touched extensively in that area by strangers remains in the body senses. How is your child going to know when not to let someone near or to say that it is not OK for someone to touch them there or anywhere else? In fact, the act of personal touch is an unconscious invitation for the body to be exposed to other people doing the same. It's like opening a door. Just be mindful of always using a sponge or a soft baby fabric for cleansing their private parts and their body.

Violations towards your baby

I've-experienced a similar problem when an adult was very rough with my one month old newborn. My baby might have seemed like a sturdy baby, but handling and rough playing with him like a 4 year old is just too early at one month. He was crying extensively, but the person did not mind his emotions. Besides, it was with an intention to provoke him for his "stubborn character". This repeated itself at 7 months and at 1,5 years old. Obviously it made him cry, not smile on any of those or other occasions. He was bothered, crying and trying to protect himself. I felt assaulted as a young mother. Again, I didn't express myself firmly: "don't touch my baby like that." I left space and time for the other adult to discover that the rough touch was not proper for neither the baby, nor for me as a mother.

Adults need to respect the mothers as an extension of their baby or child and ask for approval, just like a dogs and their owners on the street. In the end, the mother is there to protect her child and she knows her baby the best. She needs to be the confident caretaker. As an outsider you can be worried about the baby's wellbeing, or dislike his character, and therefore you are asked to ask about your concerns without being attached to the result. If you witness violence towards the baby or child, you can certainly be worried for the wellbeing of the child and the overworked and stressed mother. You should be protective. It's likely

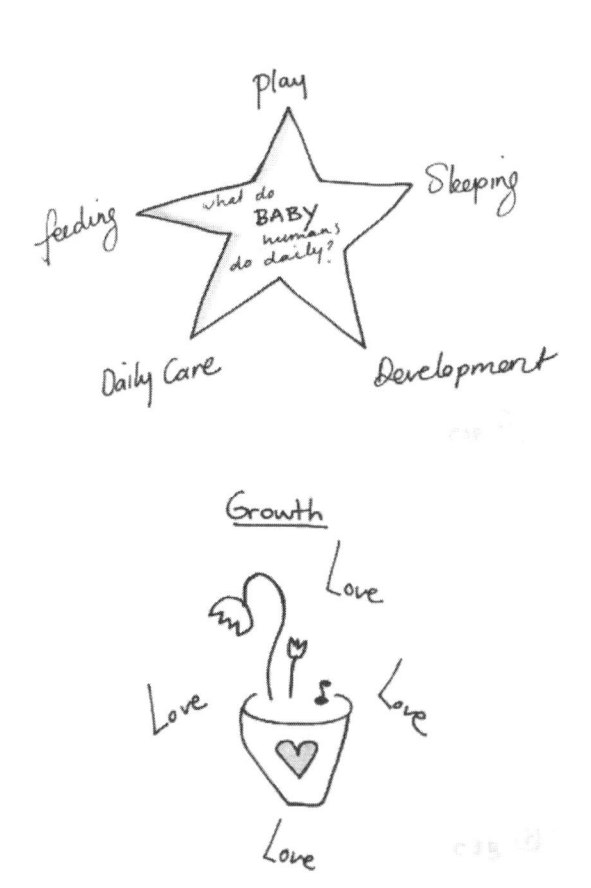

Diagram: A star labeled "what do BABY humans do daily?" with points labeled: play, Sleeping, Development, Daily Care, feeding

Diagram: A potted plant with a heart on the pot, surrounded by the words: Growth, Love, Love, Love, Love

that the mother or the father will use violence when they are overworked and overstressed, because they have reached frustration limits and they could be learning to grow their patience and non-violence in the communication with themselves, their children, their partner and the concept of 'discipline'.

A mother will need a time-out to count to ten and take a break from the routine. If the parent is continuously on this path of violence, handling from an emotional or authoritative position, a change is needed in the perceptions, attitudes and roles. We can call violence an attitude and a 'thinking' rather than a parenting skill. It is not something emotionally intelligent. Violence is negativity. Violence is from a place of weakness, even if it doesn't seem so. It is not empowering for the child nor the parent. Further education and anger management are required for the parent to strengthen their self-esteem, their sense of worth, their parental guidance and many other psychology and practical scheduling with the kids.

At some point a mother (to be) will be fearful about something that is happening to her or the wellbeing of her baby. If she receives no reassurance or support, she will experience a huge amount of stress. She's incapable of feeling safe herself and keeping her baby safe. This can be any moment before, during or after delivery of her baby. Stress brings forth the fight, flight or freeze reaction in our survival brain and our body will respond to that fight, flight or freeze reaction. Our body will not always respond though, because our mind is in the way. The fight is not actual fighting. The flight is not actual fleeing. The freeze is not actual standing still. Our brain has developed since the reptilian or prehistoric brain, it will still have these survival reactions, unless in great physical danger, it will not respond in that way.

The response of the body is through a muscle contraction and an emotion. The emotion is stored in our bodies (there is more than only the physical body) by storing the memory in our muscles, in the water of our body, in the subconscious, the brainstem, the chakras and so on. This only happens in a traumatic way when an emotion was overpowering. When we cannot process the emotion on the spot or in the close context, it will nestle behind a port of fear. The port of fear will keep it locked away as long as possible. Basically, you will remain in either the fight, flight or freeze position until you have opened the port and let out the original feeling.

Stress will either be expressed physically, emotionally, mentally, spiritually or on all four levels and will intensify if we start covering it up by 'acting normal'. A birthing woman is in an extremely vulnerable position on all these levels. She will not usually be able to execute control or self-control as easily. She is opening up to birth and this comes with a lot of internal power as well as a lot of loss on external behavior, stimuli, safety settings and reactions. She probably feels the most vulnerable in the last trimester of her pregnancy as well as the months after her body has birthed, notably with her newborn in her arms. This vulnerability grows, intensifies and can last for months and years to come.

A violation is only defined by the person themselves, no matter how you look at it from the outside. Even if a treatment was given with success and there were no bad intentions. Even if all the doctor is doing is assisting the woman and her body with birthing the baby. Only she will know if she was violated. The same applies to your baby, even without bad intentions, whenever you touch your baby's body you best ask your baby for approval. You might not have had the bad intention, but your baby will still feel violated if you cross boundaries. The great thing about babies is that they will cry it out immediately. Crying therefor is something to respond to in the moment and not to be surpassed. If you can manage this on at least 85% of the occasions, you are setting the right example on the majority of daily feeding, dressing, bathing and such.

There will likely be some crying when going into the carseat, but it is quite an obligation for their safety to be in a carseat. All the other actions during the day are not required on the moment you want them to sleep or eat or play, even if you as a parent think they 'should' be doing that and that you 'should' force them to do it. When you are parenting aware and consciously, you will only have 15% of real resistance during a week. When there is 15% real resistance you can work with that resistance by going through the "tea and talk". Slow down, hit the pause button, connect with your baby, bond with them, talk with them as if you are having tea and talk about 'your lesson' with them. Tell them what you are observing and why you think it would be a healthy choice if they went for some kind of eating, sleeping, resting, playing, activity, dressing up, dressing down, hygiene habit. Whatever it is, talk about it in a slowed down moment when your child is receptive for having a two-way conversation. And yes, it is possible in the first year and it will become a requirement in the second year to discuss their habits, rituals and routines.

The Power of NO

At each birthday toddlers hit a huge milestone, it will show up either a couple months before their birthday as well as after the date. At one year old they start saying "no", which means that they are practicing to say "no". NO is a very useful word to ward off people, to decide on what to want, to develop the willpower, to execute their own willpower and voice. Do not limit the power of "NO".

Even from the first day, the intentions you have for your child are felt and what you are doing to the body is what you are doing to the persona. There is literally no age for it. The same counts for an elderly person. Do you want to overpower them? Then they will feel overpowered. Do you want to teach them how to feel overpowered? Start overpowering them now and they will feel exactly that for the rest of their lives. Do you want to neglect or ignore your child? Then the person will feel neglected and ignored for the rest of their lives. Do you want to teach them to feel neglected and ignored? Than you should start young; start neglecting and ignoring now. I know I have experience neglect and ignorance at the height by the time I was birthing, because this is what I was taught from a very young age. It truly is quite simple, yet so complicated for us humans to comprehend. What we inflict, is what we inflict. Now start thinking about what you want to inflict, and what you do not want to inflict. Instead of thinking how your are going to master your child, let your child be their own master. Self-control in the right place is more powerful and empowering. They are the ones to control their body, behavior, hunger, thirst, hygiene, play, friendships, family, intelligence and so on. What age is the right age for that? I would say Day 0.

Birth Rights

Autonomy over ones body and to be involved in the decision-making is a birth right. Being informed on the routines, that's what consciousness is all about. Respecting the human being for being his body and having ownership of the 'body temple where the soul resides'. So even the smallest routines, from a doctor, from a nurse or from a family member should be with the utmost respect and consensus. And for the parent assisting his child in life, this mentality will help for both individuals, parent and child, being equally respected. To be respected as humans and soul beings traveling though this human experience, is the biggest gift we can give and receive. This way your baby and your growing child has a chance of growing up feeling complete, whole and respected from the inside and out. This will change our society. This will make it whole again.

Sleep Deprivation And Emotional Safety

Abandoning a woman's or man's right to feeling emotionally safe is never OK. Emotional safety is what we all want. We want to feel emotional safe in our bodies, our mind, our soul, our lives and in situations that require emotional or physical safety. Even in an emergency, there is the possibility of communicating effectively to reduce the anxiety of violation and the extreme vulnerability of a child or (pregnant) mother. Sleep deprivation is one of those situations where physical and emotional wellbeing is endangered.

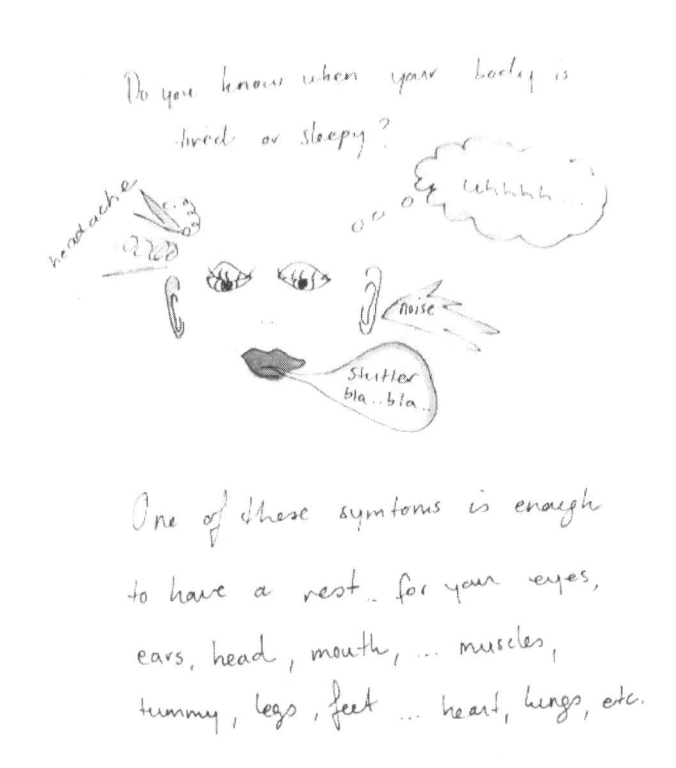

Do you know when your body is tired or sleepy?

headache... zzz... ohhhh... uhhhh... noise... Shutter bla..bla..

One of these symtoms is enough to have a rest. for your eyes, ears, head, mouth, ... muscles, tummy, legs, feet ... heart, lungs, etc.

Sleep deprivation is used in prisons as a form of torture. When mothers don't get a minimum of sleep, we are literally torturing mothers. Modern-day motherhood has become a prison to many mothers with sleepless babies or children. Unfortunately it's as much a physical prison as it is a psychological prison, because no mother will accept help in order for her to catch up on sleep. This is the biggest guilt trip we could have. So, God help us women. Men, you can be the key to our healing of our male ego - "I'm so strong! I can do this! I can do it all.". Give us the chance to be women, the chance to rest, let us be, let us relax on our own and away from everybody. Her sanity is also your sanity. And you are the only person that can really give her the big push she needs to get out of the house or into her bed, to see her friends or to do whatever is most needed to heal.

Warning: sleep deprivation can lead to serious depression, chemical imbalance, mental disease ("craziness") and even suicide.

Your birth and your mother's story

Every birth has its own story; a birth story. It can be full of joy, laughter, peace, encouragement, but it can also be full of fear, worries and even aggression. It might be a mix. The events of getting to the hospital, the contractions, the hospital experience, the pushing, the doctors, the long hours of waiting or the rush of it, it is all part of the birth story. The father of the baby might have been there, he might

Divine Powers

not have been there. He might have been too late, after baby was born, which happens for any kind of reason. Or he was eating from a bag of chips and joking around like a clown as one of my clients used to tell me. You could be dealing with an angry or afraid husband such as I've experienced myself. Everything is possible and there will always be a woman that can tell you the story of it.

Ask you mother about your birth and your grandmother about the birth of your mother. Write down the stories, as you will probably forget the details onwards. By writing it down, your mind can fit puzzle pieces together to figure out your life patterns and those of others and grow more and more into your consciousness. You can also pass the written stories on to your daughter, daughter-in law or your son's partner for clarification of their heritage. If you can, do the same on your partner's side of the women, you are providing them with valuable information. It might give you insights on your life and your relatives! Your birth story tells your life. There are books on this specific subject and it is worth digging through. We all carry our birth as a traumatic event and it might evolve your life to a better place when you have healed from it.

Dharma v.s. Karma

There is no ideal birth and you can prepare, but a plan usually does not go by plan the moment we become parents. Making some decisions is necessary and a plan can help set the intentions for it to unfold like you have intended. The intentions should describe the overall feelings and results and not so much the way that it comes about. This is the secret to conceptualizing your future birth, your general future and your future events by focusing on the result of them not by matter of facts, but by the feelings, experience or consciousness you have gained. It is somewhat related to the Law Of Attraction and the Universal Laws.

If there are no intentions, it will be Karma that decides and usually that can turn negative on you and create drama in the moment. This is not an easy exercise or skill, but perhaps you can become accustomed to it by making it a daily challenge for the next 28 days. In the online world of self-coaching individuals have named this the create28 challenge, which is a commitment to creating something related to your creativity for 28 days. Why this number? The brain needs 21-30 days in order to create a habit of something. After that month it will become a more natural thing to do, and as time passes it becomes a more automated habit until it becomes a subconscious habit. So instead of wanting to delete a bad or negative habit which you cannot control anymore because it is in your subconscious, you can replace it by a good or positive habit which will replace the negative one when practiced for 28 days. This now, is called Dharma. Quite the opposite of Karma and much more in line with the natural and universal laws of energy. Keep the focus, keep the goals, keep busy, keep creating.

To keep yourself accountable it is important to share this 'creation of the day' with other people which could be as simple as an online media such as Facebook, Instagram, a blog, Twitter or wherever you have followers.

Not having a plan goes for the hours up to actual birth and beyond. For the rest of your lives we live in the complicated zone of being a family. A unit of three or more individuals that become as one. One effects the other and they cannot live apart without being somehow affected. But how are you going to deal with this? What is your family planning? What should you think of whilst 'family planning'? These are questions to come back to and they can be dealt with when your baby reaches his First Birthday. Back to birth: as long as you keep communicating, you can or will have the chance to feel safe and supported by someone. Through your communication and intention of having the most positive birth, you can actually create this result and reach this target consciously and unconsciously. In best cases the birth is a positive, very positive or extremely positive experience depending on the people you encounter, and the way you feel about the feedback you are getting or any personal sensations.

Talking with your mother about her birth story birthing you, can heal your relationship if there have been parts of the birth broken or overstressed. Focus on forgiveness, recognition and acceptance. Forgiveness is given by 'giving the forGIVEness, forth or before anything else'. It is a deep kept secret or perhaps a misinterpreted act in the churches. Forgiveness, even if the other person is not physically part of it, is your key to becoming one with yourself. One with yourself means that you will find the grounds of safety where you were once born from, the source of consciousness. These grounds feel like the vast ocean grounds where no waves of emotion exist or the vast sky where you can breath forever freely. It is a great place to be, because you are not riding the tireless waves or the constant hurricanes on the ocean of life. Or whatever imagination you feel your inner life is taking you for. Forgiveness for others and self, it will set you free, free from others and free from yourself. This also works on a level of society and world. You can do this in a coaching session and this you can make into a Create28 Challenge. I would love to see it online and I might even start doing it myself.

The Aftermath

You might want to prepare for the aftermath of birth. I don't like to label women as "postnatal depressed" or "hormonal", because it seems an insult that strangers make in order to put a woman down, denigrate her and give an excuse to their own intrusive, rude or insulting behavior and thoughts. A very typical excuse. On the other hand, we all seem to expect that a woman acts "normal" especially now that the baby is "out". And that she is physically able to carry on with her every day tasks plus some. Her chores and missions, especially keeping up everyone else's agenda, have maximized after giving birth. This makes me angry and worried, because we are not meant to live non-tribal, especially at these years of early childhood.

We are scarring women (and children and men), damaging them and with them our world. No-one grows up sanely if they are not surrounded by a community. If we live individually, we should at least be able to compensate the safety network, services and family ties. Who decided to lose this important role of community and motherhood? Not all societies expect women to be up on their feet and acting "normal" within the first month or months. In Bahrain and other Asian countries there are the "40 sacred days" where a woman is taken care of and is supposed to rest as much as possible. In some European countries the maternity leave covers 1-3 years for both mother and father. Basically, they give women a long maternity leave or they surround the women with a circle of other women to support her. These settings are the most ideal (the second one being more ideal) and something that we should perhaps seek for if we are aware of the aftermath of birth.

In the Middle-East women are supported by cleaning maids and nannies, which does not cover the scala of requirements, but at least she is not isolated and on her own. In other countries there are mothers or mother-in-laws that are supportive the first weeks or months, yet it does not cover all the needs. With a lot of budget planning or extra expenses, even in West-European countries, you can hire many of the needs: cleaning ladies, a doula, massages at home, a nanny, meal deliveries for the quick eating, groceries delivered, cook for homemade meals, daycare for baby or toddler, extra nurses, taxi to drive around and I could probably think of more services like sleep trainers, psychologists and a parent coach. Again, this requires a bit of planning of your budget, but I believe it doesn't need to be exceptionally expensive if you pick and choose. It can be done for a period of three months, phased in and out, but it needs to be booked and planned in your Third Trimester before birth sets in.

Your sanity and health are worth it, that is for sure. Who cares if your family is fed from full meal deliveries or a home cook? You could also make a deal with a restaurant to give you a discount for three months of healthy meals. Our culture will tell us that it is "not done" and a "luxury", but I would call it "survival", "necessity" and "helping each other out".

How to support PPD

Because postpartum situations are not always our own choice, we have to look for alternatives. If possible, you can create this network of a sisterhood or 'Framily'. You can invest in hiring the nurses and housemaids or ask your own family to be a specific, intensive support for long duration with a phase in and phase out. Stubborn as I am, I did none with my second baby. Instead I moved countries, so don't take me as a great example. Be more wise, be less stubborn. Be less "Strong" for that matter. We are not meant to be economic and put out male energy, especially pregnant and unpregnant. Perhaps this is where the actual depression carries its roots! We cannot truly be a mothering mother after giving birth. We are missing our 'sisters' and forced to household chores and day time duties or jobs when we are still bound to nurture our baby, body and soul.

Placenta pills can support in PSTD and healing your birth story. Placenta pills are taken from your own placenta and dried in a complete safe method into capsules. You need to decide on this in the third trimester so you can arrange the certified placenta pill maker to pick up your placenta in the hours after birth. Also you need your hospital to co-operate in keeping a piece of the placenta. Realizing after my second, not first, baby that depression is a natural occurrence after birth, I would definitely prevent or sooth this phase by having the placenta pills. Another option with the placenta is to have homeopathic pills made by the same company. These are meant for baby whenever they are going through stress or disease. Possibly it aids in healing serious disease. With my next baby I would also make sure to store the stem cells from the umbilical cord in case they suffer from a serious disease. Don't forget: when the baby has pushed his way out, let the umbilical cord pulse for one minute until it is done pulsing. These are your babies super nutritions and immunity.

Birth trauma: the final say

On a deeper level there is the experience and the theory that when we are about to give birth to our baby, we recreate what our own mothers experienced with us unconsciously. These traumas can pass on for the next generations, usually in a cycle of seven generations, where the seventh has a chance to break the patterns.

The mother's patterns can be repeated until you realize the mind-body connection and release or replace the pattern with a new one. In preparing for your upcoming pregnancy it would be optimal for you to experience a re-birthing session with a Re-Birth Healer. I didn't have the courage to do this. I can see the benefit for our own lives and the mirror that our children are in that what we pass on in a positive and negative way. More than ever, I can see how my four year old is a pure extension of my happiness and unhappiness. It is my duty to make him happy. Our children take with them the unfinished story that we have given them. In that sense, I feel regret not taking even better care of some unresolved anger issues and naturally I worry now about my child's inner world. Worry comes easily to parents with a bad conscious!

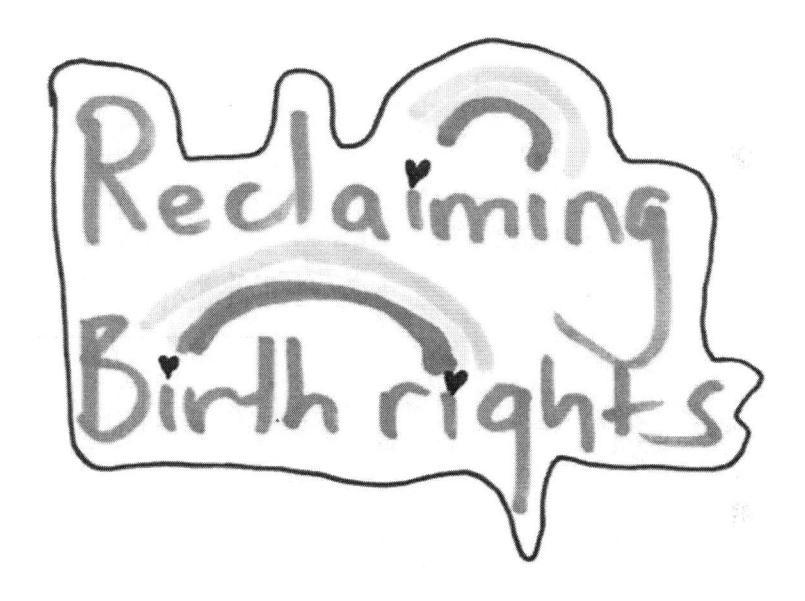

Reclaiming Birth rights

Worry and guilt comes easily to parents with a bad conscious! Clear your conscious, stay clean.

- Andromeda L.C.

How to recover from Birth Trauma

There can be four and possibly more steps to solving Birth Trauma:

1. Transformational Breath Work: to start learning to breathe simply and more deeply. The majority of people breath through their upper chest instead of with "the belly" or the pulling down of the diaphragm. This is an effect and a cause of mental stress.

2. Rebirth sessions within a group setting: These sessions are often a single session focused on the birthing moment and experience. The group is brought to a trance where the body relives the experience and also has a chance to release any stuck emotions. The councillor will guide you on this journey.

3. Inner Child Therapy: This is not focused on the birth experience, but heals part of our lives in the Early Childhood.

4. Water Re-Birthing: This is a private session. You will be taken in a pool or a hot tub and with the guidance of a Re-Birth Healer, you will start to release cellular memories in your own DNA of the Birth Trauma.

It is wonderful to feel complete with a new baby, but no one here on earth is here to complete you. This is your job: Wholeness comes from within and it is there in the 'lost and found' to be found. First you get lost, then you get found. The more you accept this as a truth, the better you will not be placing unrealistic expectations on your child or your partner, your parents or even yourself. When your parent does not recognise and accept and embrace your essential being as a child, actually the extension of themselves, you will create a "wishful personality" within the first five to six years of life. In psychology this is called a "persona". You are by these means separated from your natural, essential being. A wishful personality, is not a wishful personality at all.

The beliefs you have about your own 'self', your persona, are less than perfect. You feel weakened. You feel unaccepted. You feel unloved. You feel unresolved. You feel incomplete. You might feel shame or insecurity as a result of it. You might not even feel like you were ever born into this world! I know this exact feeling all too well.

Surely, we have to keep on living, so you develop strategies to cope with this incompleteness. And in coping with your lost self, you will find difficulties in the connection with others. Unfortunately, it's extremely hard to be aware of your difficulties, because you don't have a counter experience or the right kind of example or reference to compare 'yourself' with. You can compare yourself with the self of yesterday or many years ago. There might have been pivotal points of change in your inner self. You felt stronger, more whole, more complete, more competent, more at ease in your own skin and more at peace with life.

Perhaps you avoid the good experiences all together or cut them short. Do you want to be unhappy and miserable? No, deep down you don't, but you do not know what happiness and love is, so you are looking for anything that will make you feel something. And usually that something is pain. Pain is a more direct and accessible feeling than happiness, joy, love, humor, success. So your initial self is found in the connection with people and in particular your romantic, intimate relationship. Wether it be positive or negative interactions. The question is: which side will win? Your happiness or your persona?

No guarantees in life

As a parent of whatever type, I have no guarantee over my child's inner world. I'm as strong, as weak, as perfect, as imperfect, as human, as inhuman, as any parent. No I am not cruel. That I'm conscious about. I am 100% human. More than you, as a conscious parent. That is the only guarantee I have. As a matter of fact I don't have a full scope on how much I've been healed, especially in relationship to how my children are affected. I have an idea of my own consciousness and how conscious I am in my unconsciousness. I have a slighter idea on how I am affecting and hurting my child and their future inner child. All I know is that I've gone through spiritual enlightenment possibly by revisiting my childhood, the current parenthood and the persona as well as marriage. I see the world differently. I see it as it is in hell and as it is in heaven. I feel enlightened. I found peace.

I'm dealing with the relationship with my children through conscious parenting principles which are completely "owned" by me because I live what I believe (be-live), I walk the talk and talk the walk. I feel totally empowered in parenting. What I do need, is a balance in my time spent with my kids and some hours away from the kids, which unfortunately has not been the case for the past years and as of yet. For other mothers and fathers it could have been the other way round and you might feel the guilt weighing on you. When I get overworked, with kids and life, I start to lose my cool and I need to get out of the house from time to time to remain less wild and bewildered. As any job, we need a break from our routine to refuel our batteries and our clear out our mind. Being a parent is intense, no matter how you divide your time. For your kids to be a true joy, you need to find your own joy and see and create the joy in them, with them.

Becoming your original self

The original child is filled with life, open, spontaneous and receptive, but whilst being a child, he or she is dependant and helpless towards adult beings. The original adult is independent and helpful, but they so often suffer from the dependency and helplessness towards their inner child and therefore other adults and "the World". The question is; how can we become mature again? How can we again feel filled with life, open, spontaneous and receptive?

Adults:

- feel lonely
- feel abandoned
- feel attention deficit
- feel pressured
- feel they are a failure
- feel they need to perform

- feel they are emotionally overwhelmed
- feel they are numb
- feel like they don't know how to deal,.. with life, others or themselves.

These patterns keep repeating, over and over and over and over, until we break lose and move into consciousness as a home. The moment we wake up to our adult self and start freeing our inner child from past wounds and current emotions, we start our healing journey.

As the inner child grows into more independence, the adult grows into more wholeness. The child is welcomed back into wholeness and guided by his new parent: YOU. That is the greatness of it; you get to parent your own child from now on. This is also conscious parenting.

You are fully capable, powerful and willing to be whole and to be your own parent. You are an adult now and that is what being adult means! Parent yourself. Use Conscious Parenting; it is meant for you more than anyone else. Your children will profit from it most directly without having to apply any other 'technique'. And when you are a

To do list

Conscious Parent, your partner and everyone ready to be part of a positive life will profit from it too.

One such therapy for meeting the inner child is named Neo-Hypnotherapy or Hypnotherapy and it addresses all the feelings, images, voices and memories from the past that

Sleep

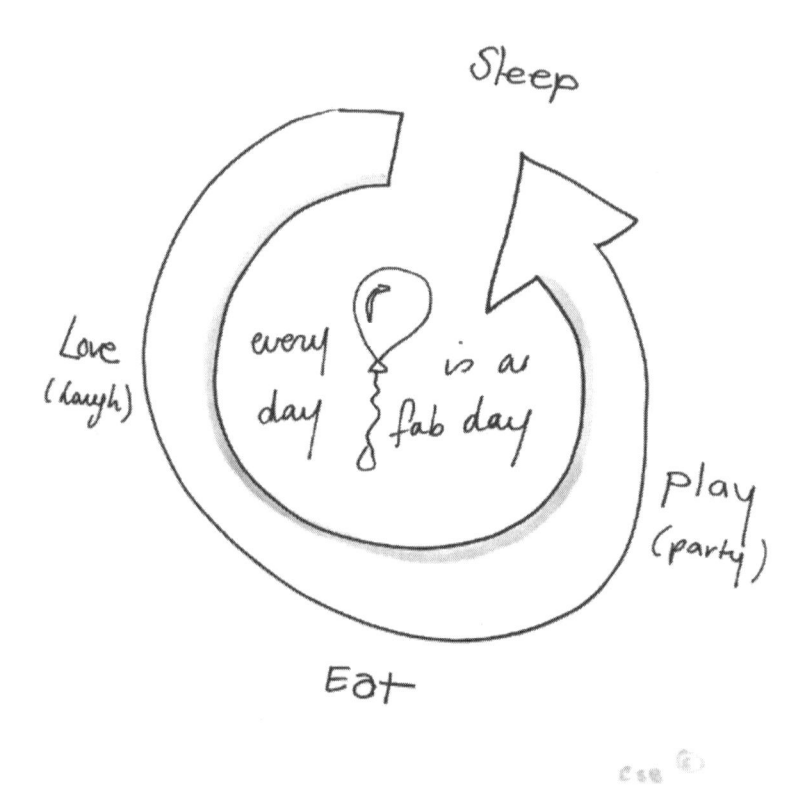

Love (laugh)

every day is a fab day

Play (party)

Eat

need healing. Timeline healing can be part of this technique or the therapist might work with miasmas and the Akashic Records. Healing is;

- awareness
- acceptance or forgiveness of the other
- forgiveness or rather "making it whole"
- letting go
- rewriting your story for a new, positive direction

Marry yourself

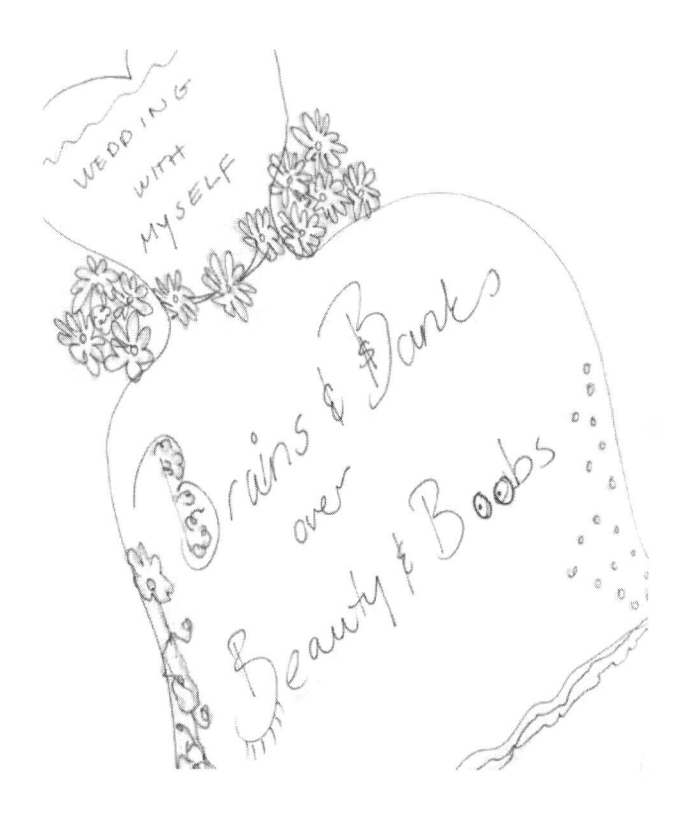

Another therapy for addressing the persona (or personas) and making the adult become its original and whole self is Voice Dialogue; a psychotherapy from the seventies and quite popular with new therapists because it is easily accessible. You will simulate different selfs and through this discovery and self talk, you will learn to heal and bring back yourself to one person. We constantly have parts of ourselves floating in the universe and in the ties with people from our current day and the past. The personas are trying to defend you, survive you and make you feel "not hurt", to feel "whole". In reality they are not empowering, they are weakening you and pushing the original you to the background. They are merely a mirage of the real (part of) you that needs healing and needs to settle back into your body and mind. Not (capable of) being you is what hurts us humans the most. Fear is our prison. I call back all my aspects home, now, and so it is, welcome them back home. Say it out loud.

Another way of putting things is; our body has been built through cells and stimulation, through pregnancy and birth. With the "wrong" stimulation - inherent to human existence - our body is than expressed in the "wrong" way. Responding to the initial stimulation in the cells and the nervous system was coloured and effected by Birth Trauma. Our nervous system is a big complex and takes up a big role in the healing process of a healthy body-mind connection. In the current day, your body is still reacting and expressing itself through this initial "wrong" information and stimulation. Through consciousness, meditation and therapy we can find ourselves in the womb of the Universe and Mother Earth which supports us in the most perfect way and presentation. Mother Earth, Gaia, is our true mother. We will feel carried by peace. The body's intelligence and healing capabilities are activated when Father Peace enters those parts of lives most effected. True and spontaneous healing, even of the physical body, can take place at this moment.

Other therapies related to Birth Trauma:

Jungian, Psychodrama, Transactional Analysis, NLP, Gestalt, Psychosynthese, Client Centered Therapy, Mindfulness, Enneagram, Gurdjief-filosofie, Retrievement of aspects, Sjamanism, Rebirthing, Breath Work, Body Work, Anger Management, Stress Management, Conflict Management, Meditation, Yoga, Somatic Experience, Chakra balancing, NES Health Therapy and more ...

Consider and research these therapies when you encounter real disease, discomfort and difficulties within yourself or your children.

Until now parenting has been a fashion, not a science. More and more science is done on the physical and developmental baby. One day parenting will be a science. New parents will always search for the equilibrium between routine (what parents want) and bonding (what babies want). Let us see what the science and society of tomorrow says about this equilibrium.

We don't become Mother overnight

Let's say, with your first baby, you become a "Mommy"; it is like a young, rookie, mother. With time and experience, like any job, we become more and more senior. So from mommy we grow ourselves and our organization into a "Mom" or "Mother".

As we continuously push ourselves and develop to the better version of ourselves for our children, we become a real Mother. Not all mothers make it to the title Mother. They have lost themselves or the connection with their child along the way. They decided to separate from the family or they became mentally or emotionally sick and abusive. Some mothers did not succeed in healing themselves or their families and have fallen into a sickness or a mental illness that separates them from themselves and their children. These are mothers either out of the picture, alcoholic, abusive, "sick" or involved in something truly painful.

When we have succeeded in becoming a Mother we have the chance to become a Grandmother. A Grandmother is someone that has the best intentions for children of the next generation. Not necessarily her own grandchildren. A mother does not need her own children to become a mother in her life or the community. A mother is a role and a heart for the living and the expressions of it. This system is a first introduction into a rewritten chakra system and how we evolve or achieve an Inner Lotus status or en-lightenment of our lives. I will explain this cycle more and how to live it outside of this book.

We need to be present and connected with the right intentions to wear the crown of the grandmother type; the crone. After Grandmother, we have the chance to become concerned with the world and the passing on of wisdom. If she reached self healing she incarnates into a Crone. We can become Crone without ever having had our own children. So, like any other career, these titles grow with time, experience and motivation. In this sense, we cannot expect a mommy with 1 or 2 years experience to be expressing herself and her life as a Mother or Grandmother. Give her some damn slack! She just came from being a Maiden, the initial adulthood of a Woman.

LOTUS & CHAKRA SYSTEM

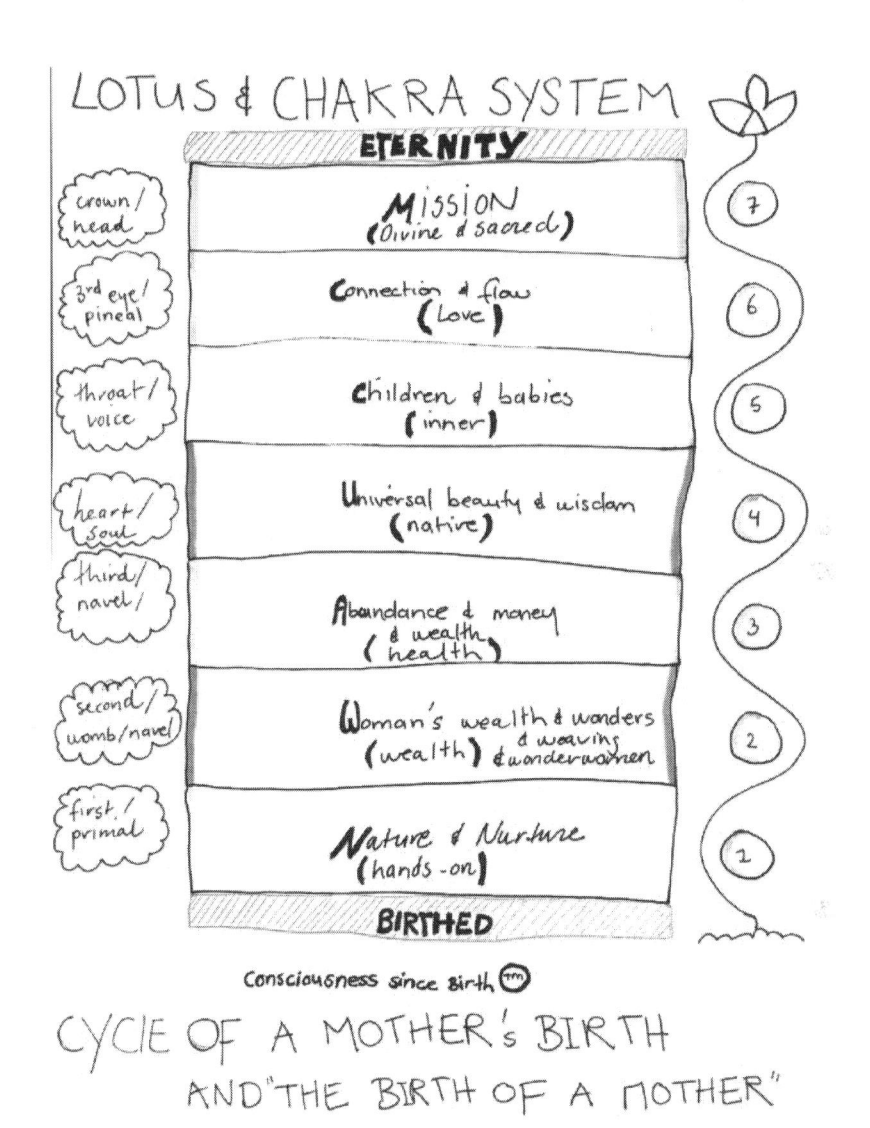

ETERNITY

Chakra location	Theme	#
crown/head	Mission (Divine & sacred)	7
3rd eye/pineal	Connection & flow (Love)	6
throat/voice	Children & babies (inner)	5
heart/soul	Universal beauty & wisdom (native)	4
third/navel	Abundance & money & wealth (health)	3
second/womb/navel	Woman's wealth & wonders & weaving (wealth) & wonderwomen	2
first/primal	Nature & Nurture (hands-on)	1

BIRTHED

Consciousness since birth ™

CYCLE OF A MOTHER'S BIRTH AND "THE BIRTH OF A MOTHER"

We don't become Father overnight

As we don't become a mother overnight, we don't become a father overnight. Fathers usually will need more time to find the bond with the baby and to find their role and responsibility towards baby, wife and family. Most men are afraid of such a fragile, vulnerable baby being. The bonding is often stood in the way or not stimulated by the mother. Or the father might be seen as a softy if he is over involved with their baby or children. A good idea is to start with "parent - child date" as early on. Even a "sibling date".is a good idea, of course accompanied by a parent or guardian. On such a date the two individuals have a chance to encounter each other, talk and create memories. This is the quality time we need in order to create a strong bond amongst the members of the family, just like "family time". On these dates, the father has a chance to bond with the baby or child, no matter how young. And to see the world through the eyes of the father instead of absent provider. For boys the 'boy time' is vital to the growth of the male persona. In the 1970's, when the tribal concept revived, the parenting acknowledged the importance of men spending time with men. This was certainly not the case in the 1950's where dad was considered absent.

Overall, the father has a vital, crucial role to both boy and girl children. Girl's grow their confidence and their womanhood through the interaction and perception of the father. They become strong, whole women that know about a loving relationship. When they missed their father or father role as such a present and alive component, they tend to lack self-esteem and seek their esteem from the wrong type of men or friends. In other words: absent or abusive men and friends. When the woman is whole and has a reference of love, she will imitate this relationship in her intimate relationships with men and women alike.

Getting through the Marriage

For an effective marriage and parenting after children I would advice to at least think and act upon Marriage Counseling before marriage and before having or conceiving the baby. You can do counseling separately and together, depending on the agenda and type of counseling. If there are no problems to solve, there is more inclination to sit together on being informed on marriage and Parent Effectiveness. If there are problems, individually or with the couple, you are more inclined to sit separately and solve issues internally before talking to your partner in a dialogue. My advice is to go back to the moment where you

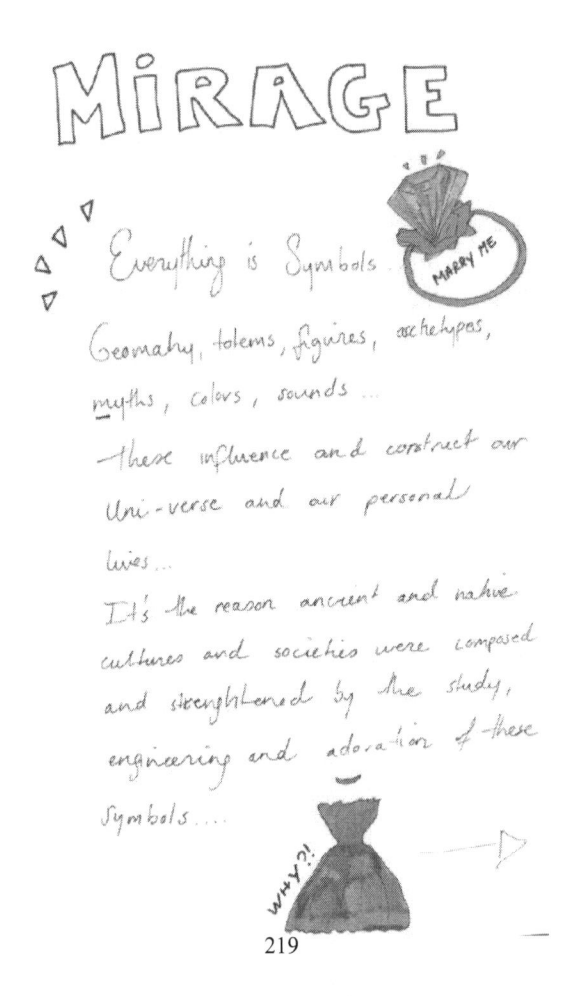

MIRAGE

Everything is Symbols... MARRY ME

Geomancy, totems, figures, archetypes, myths, colors, sounds...

—these influence and construct our Uni-verse and our personal lives...

It's the reason ancient and native cultures and societies were composed and strenghtened by the study, engineering and adoration of these Symbols....

WHY?!

felt the most hurt inflicted by your partner. This was the moment you had a misunderstanding, even if you had been hurt and disappointed in the past. Of course, the question should be if you should continue with the present relationship if the foundation is based on a lack of love, understanding, respect and connection.

Parenting workshops are extremely effective before baby and as followup in the first year. Both the father and the mother in the couple will see other fathers and mothers struggling with the same issues, which can actually bond the couple for a good cause. Another two powerful group sessions amongst the self-help for couples and families are Shadow -Light Retreats and Family Constellations.

Alchemy and Nature Religions

Both Nature Religions and Alchemy hold ancient tools to help us on unconscious levels in order to bring forth our consciousness into existence and into the light. Symbols, plants, stones, words (mantras) and rituals are vibrational tools that heal the dark, the wounded, the shadow of ourselves and that push us into the light, into the higher frequency and into the love. There are many people knowledgable about these practices that have gone through this process and that will shift your consciousness and give you the tools through a direct conversation, contact and session. Once you have learnt from their words of wisdom, their sessions, books and such, you have a reference to work with in your own spiritual practice. You will remember intuitively and start downloading your own legacies and inheritance.

Sitting or standing with yourself in the moment, where you have hit the pause button and continue to pause the button long enough, are moments of clarity. Seek those moments of slowing down the time, stretching the minutes and dropping into existence for moments of clarity. As soon as the mind jumps, go back into the position you were previously and continue your session of silence and clarity. These are the moments with answers and guidance from our higher selves, whatever that might mean to you. The more you are mindful, connected and living in the now, the more your daily habits and work will become mindful, connected and powerful. This is what we call meditation. So meditation can literally be any two minutes of the day, even whilst playing with your children or doing a chore. It is also a great moment before starting an activity or when ending an activity.

When we are in touch with the consciousness of the moment, we can follow that instinct or intuition. It might be to click a certain page, open a certain profile or go to a certain store. It's that one crazy thought, inspiration or motivation you have, no matter how general, meaningless or simple it might seem. The more you do this in your home and outside of your home, the more you fall into the synchronicity of your life. Do not hold yourself back and let yourself be guided. Even by your children's intuition and inspiration. The universe talks through the actions of your children to guide you to the light and purpose of your life, whilst keeping you away from dangers and daily mishaps. You will find synchronicity by following their intentions rather than your own because you are governed mostly by your mind. They will show you that one missing idea or puzzle piece to continue your day, week, month and year in a purposeful, meaningful manner. It is for you to act upon and I know you will find a thousand opportunities for an exhilarating life.

The Mother wound and Phantom Mothers

We tend to think we are always loved, even if we were not. We tend to think this, even if we were abused, molested or taken on a ride of manipulation and neglect. Welcome to the phantom mother; she is there, but not really. She might even be a type of poltergeist.

We refuse to think that perhaps we were not loved. If we were loved, would we still feel miserable as adults? Perhaps, yes. If we were loved, would we know better what to do with ourselves and our life? If we were loved, would we want to revenge on other people and cause harm in unhealthy relationships? If we were loved, would we not feel great and capable most of the time?

Sons have been trained and are expected to be protective of their mother and her feelings, sometimes at all costs. Even the mother wound and the drama in their lives are protected this way. Sons will not marry a woman or wait well into their forties, because their mother does not accept another woman in their lives. And they do not mind to continue making their son's life miserable with her misery, authority and control.

The problem is that our mothers were not loved. And as they were not loved, they do not love us enough. As all parents or humans; they look and feel through their own pair of glasses. The broken ones. This in return creates the Mother wound. Some mother wounds are bigger than others. Some mothers inflicted more sorrow on different levels of life, being, love. They could have been neglect, over involved or suffocating. They could have been the abuser or the stander by. They could have been perfectly normal and yet you feel perfectly abnormal. The Mother wound is in each one of us. Just like the birth trauma. Healing the mother wound is of great importance to both women and men. Men were also born from a wounded mother and were unloved. Women will regain their feminine power and sovereignty. Men will regain their feminine capabilities and respect for the feminine. If you could or cannot respect your mother, why would you respect women in general? If you could or cannot respect your mother, why would you respect the mother and woman in you? Much applies to women and men, and let us not forget or misunderstand that patriarchy, domination and sex driven industries are built by women as much as men. It might very well be a woman behind the booby billboards and what to think of the entire fashion industry run by women? Women keep the culture alive, they sustain it through their own wounds and mis-use of power and creation. It is in the mother's hands to create a new world, new culture and new society.

The Mother wound is generalized. There are specific types of mothers which you might help you to categorize your mother. It helps to label or define in order to let go of it with time, when your own healing is completed. You might have had a Narcotic or Neurotic Mother; someone addicted to substances and which have bothered and affected you. It could have been cigarettes, alcohol, social media, boyfriends, hobby, fitness, t.v. or simply the mom job itself. Your mom might have been a Depressed Mother; never available, emotionally absent, pity on life, pity on herself or simply confronted with a multitude of problems. She might have been a Narcissistic Mother; someone that looks only at herself and yet lacks self-reflection and efforts toward you or the responsibilities that come with your body, mind and soul.

With the above mothers you do not or did not actually have a relationship. A relationship is a two way street with mutual love, respect and involvement. If you are together through conflict and negative feelings, you are having an entanglement. Lots of people have entanglements. Especially when we are not aware of what a good, healthy or loving relationship is and when we still need healing in order to be a whole person. When we say "opposites attract", that is perfectly fine in one way but in another way it means that two broken halves are fitting together. Ideally we have a relationship with someone that is a whole person and it is sustainable when we ourselves are whole. And do you want to be fully loved for the first time? Focus on finding the love and not the dream or romance. Finding your Twin Flame is a quest for unconditional love in a partner that can be worth the wait.

Everything about Me is about "M"

As I discovered, researched and healed the Mother wound, as much as it can be healed, I realized and still am I realizing the depth of this wound. The relationship with your mother, the way your were conceived and perceived, and if this was scarring a deep wound in you, also shapes and "makes" everything relating to you. The "ME" or "M". When I consider the power of language, I can see that all words that start with M in our lives are affected. The Mother wound effects all the other concepts and experiences starting with M's.

My-self, our Make-up, our Me-decine, our Ma-rriage, our Mate, our Money, our Memories, our Mentality, our Memes and More.

Me-decine means everything that is our healing, our talents

and our passion which we find in nature, ourself and the creations like music and the arts. Marriage is the union with your second half, wether it be your Twin Flame, Soul Mate or (Mothering) Other Half. Marriage is a name and institution that offers or can offer; stability, wholeness, justice, foundation honesty, integrity, loyalty, conscientiousness, beneficence, intelligence, totality and perfection. But only if you choose so. You can become whole through the Mar-Riage, which is your own Mirage, Rage and Mirror.

To further analyze your mother wound look into the character type analysis by psychoanalyst Wilhelm Reich and the beliefs you have around 'I am not enough'. This belief could be 'I am not pretty or handsome enough', 'I am not intelligent enough', 'I am not strong enough', 'I am not sensitive enough', 'I am not kind enough' and so forth. The mother is not only your actual mother, it is the society as a whole and how we perceive Mother Earth, Gaia and the relationship we have with Fatherly Peace. The place where you feel you are not enough, has been pushed into the shadows and it is that which you are actually thriving in. If you can let it into the light of your life, you will thrive.

Helpful websites:

www.postpartumdads.com

www.beyondtheblues.com.

www.saddaddy.com

www.parents.com

www.babycentre.co.uk

Further Reading and Research

Scientific articles and books

The "Stress" of Being Born. Hugo Lagercrantz and Theodore A. Slotkin mentioned in Scientific American, Vol. 254, No. 4, pages 100-107 (92-102); April 1986. (also 'The Good Stress of Being Born', 2016)

The Importance of "Awareness" for Understanding Fetal Pain. David J. Mellor, Tamara J. Diesch, Alistair J. Gunn and Laura Bennet mentioned in Brain Research Reviews, Vol. 49, No. 3, pages 455-471; November 2005.

The Emergence of Human Consciousness: From Fetal to Neonatal Life. Hugo Lagercrantz and Jean-Pierre Changeux mentioned in Pediatric Research, Vol. 65, No. 3, pages 255-260; March 2009.

Creativity: Flow and the Psychology of Discovery and Invention, Mihaly Csikszentmihalyi, Harper Perennial, 1996 and Flow, Mihaly Csikszentmihalyi, Harper Perennial, 1990

The Highly Sensitive Person, Helping Our Children to Thrive When The World Overwhelms them, Elaine. N. Aron PH.D, Broadway Books New York, 2002

The Middle Passage, From Misery to Meaning in Mid-Life Crisis, James Hollis, Inner City Books, 1993

Emotional Intelligence: Why It Can Matter More Than IQ, Daniel Goleman, Bantam Books, 2005 and Focus: The Hidden Driver of Excellence, Daniel Goleman, Harper Paperbacks, 2015

The Whole-Brain Child, Revolutionary Strategy To Nurture Your Child's Developing Mind, Daniel J. Siegel, M.D., and Payne Bryson, Bantam Books, 2012

Body, Soul, and Baby, A Doctor's Guide to the Complete Pregnancy Experience, from Preconception to Postpartum, Tracy W. Gaudet, M.D, Bantam Book, New York, 2007.

The Collapse of Parenting, Leonard Sax MD, PhD, Basic Books, New York, 2016

Consciousness and Personal Development

The New Earth, Awakening To Your Life's Purpose, Eckhart Tolle, Penguin Putnam Inc 2006

The Power Of Now, A Guide To Spiritual Enlightenment, Eckart Tolle, Hodder & Stoughton General Division, 2001

Life Code, The New Rules for Winning in The Real World, Dr. Phil McGraw, Bird Street Books, 2013

Designing Your Life, Bill Burnett & Dave Evans, Knopf Doubleday Publishing Group, 2016

Families and How to Survive Them, Robbin Skynner & John Cleese, Titles Distributed by Oxford University Press (Australia and New Zealand), 1984

Quand l'Amour Manque Commet se Reconstruire? Jean-Claude Liaudet, l'Archipel, Paris, 2000

Parenting, Education and Culture

Praktisch Projectmanagement, Handleiding bij het voorbereiden, realiseren en beheersen van projecten, Ten Gevers & Tjerk Zijlstra, Academic Service, Schoonhoven, 1997 (Dutch)

Dear Parent: Caring for Infants With Respect (2nd Edition), Magda Gerber, Resources for Infant Educators (RIE), 2003

Positive Discipline, Jane Nelsen, Cheryl Erwin, and Roslyn Duffy, Harmony, New York, 2015

Raising Boys, Steve Biddulph, HarperCollins UK, 2013 and The Complete Secrets of Happy Children, Steve Biddulph, HarperCollins Publishers, 2013

Secrets of the Baby Whisperer, How to Calm, Connect and Communicate, Tracy Hogg, Ballantine Books, 2001

The Conscious Parent, Transforming Ourselves Empowering Our Children, Shefali Tsabary, Namaste Publishing, 2014

Montessori from the Start: The Child at Home, from Birth to Age Three, Paula Polk Pillard and Lynn Lilard Jessen, Schocken Books, New York 2003

The Danish Way of Parenting, Jessica Joelle Alexander and Iben Sandahl, Penguin Random House LLC, New York 2016

Bringing Up Bébé: One American Mother Discovers the Wisdom of French Parenting, Pamela Druckerman, Penguin Press 2012

Online

Scientific resources:
www.birthpsychology.com APPAH Association
www.ahaparenting.com Aha Parenting
www.happiestbaby.com Dr. Karp

Conscious parenting:
www.sandrafazio.com The Conscious Parent Blog
www.jicp.ca Journey into Conscious Parenting.
www.whats-your-sign.com (Avia, on symbolism)

Natural remedies:
www.mama-natura.com (calming nerves and colics)

www.bachflowers4kids.com (calming nerves and emotions)
www.NESHealth.com (scanning and healing remedies)

International Programs
(attended by the author)

Andragogy, specialised in Dance Movement, University of Social Sciences, Hogeschool Arnhem en Nijmegen, The Netherlands 2000-2004

Core Quantum Method Hypervoyager, Gabriele Eckhart, Baarn, 2007
www.hypervoyager-cqm.de

Creative Consciousness, Masters Programs, Mark Steinberg, Belgium and The Netherlands
www.creativeconsciousness.com

NES Health, Energy For Life / Your Body Is Your Best Doctor, Peter Fraser and Harry Massey
www.neshealth.com

Consciousness Since Birth Series

I, II, III

Questions pondered in the series:

- What is Consciousness and what are the benefits for you, your child, and human kind?
- What is Conscious Parenting and how is it different from regular Parenting?
- How can we apply Consciousness and become a Conscious Parent?
- Can my child become a Conscious Child?

Consciousness Since Birth Series

I, II, III

What you get from these books:

- Seeing Yourself and Baby as a Whole Human Being,

- Taking Control and Responsibility of Your Life,

- Understanding the Nature and Nurture of Things,

- Being a Calm, Confident, Caring Communicator,

- Seeking for Belonging, Connection & Flow in the right place,

- Parenting and Daily Life Routines Come with Ease,

- Creating Your Life Consciously and Creatively,

- and Much More.

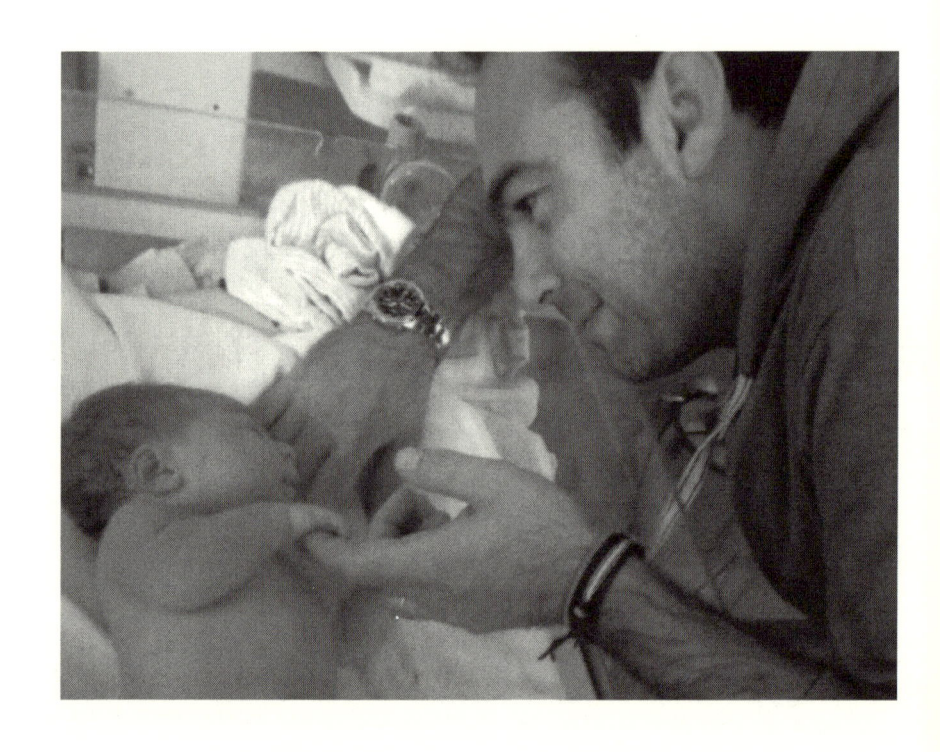

Shine Bright You Crazy Diamond

Parenting is not so much an act, as it is a being.

− Andromeda L.C.

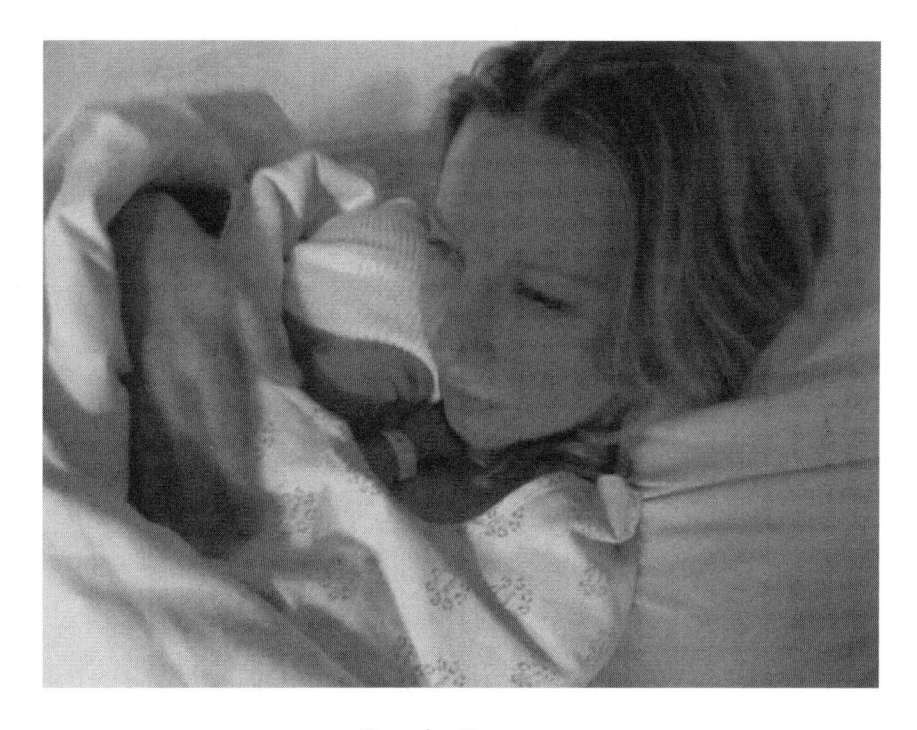

Rock On

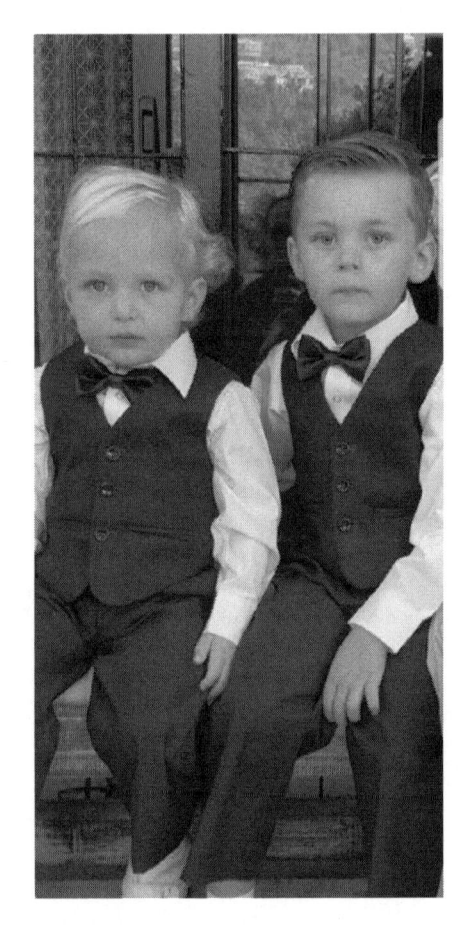

You Are Love

NOTE TO THE READERS AND PUBLISHING HOUSES:

If interested in further editing and publishing of this book, please contact the author for inquiries or a proposal. This version of the book is all rights reserved. The author has the desire to put out the information without further delay. She is looking for the investment in professional translators and a publishing house if they can provide the platform for further awareness of this book and its content on a national or international level.

Dear Reader,

If you notice any mistakes or corrections, please contact me so I can attend to it. If you would like to comment or give feedback, it would be lovely to hear from you.

Contact the Author:

Andromeda Limmen Chehab

Join the Facebook Community:

The Conscious Parents Of Mommy Life Coach

Visit www.mommylifecoachme.com for downloads

Open to calls and collaborations

Follow Instagram: @mommy_life_coach

Bahrain, Worldwide

There is no wrong or right. There is only 'what is' in you as a person and parent.

What is in you? what is your "isness"? Where do you want to go?

- Andromeda L.C.